Being Brain Healthy

Being Brain Healthy

What my recovery from brain injury taught me and how it can change your life

by
Ruth Curran, MS

Rolling Mulligan Publishing
San Diego, CA 92103

The ideas, procedures, and suggestions in this book are not intended as a substitute for the medical advice of a trained health professional. All matters regarding your health require medical supervision. Consult your physician before adopting the suggestions in this book, as well as about any condition that may require medical attention. The author and publisher disclaim any liability arising directly or indirectly from the use of the book (or of any products mentioned herein).

Being Brain Healthy
Rolling Mulligan Inc.
3410 Hawk St.
San Diego, CA 92103

ISBN 978-0692399958

*To Dan and David, who make me strong,
and in memory of Mom and Millie, who light my way.*

Contents

INTRODUCTION

Why I Am Writing This Book

I am writing this book because my experience with a brain injury and my path to Okay was not typical. I am one of the lucky ones. Although there are those who do get help and have wonderful support, and those who will walk out of the fog on to a positive path to a different but good life, that is, unfortunately, not the usual story.

By nature, medicine and treatment are made to deal with sickness. Rebuilding after a brain incident or setting yourself up to nourish your brain and grow new neurons must first be about health, well-being, and amplifying the quality of your life. It also needs to be about making those things you are already doing, and must continue doing to live successfully in the world, a vehicle or platform you can use to think and live better.

I know that was a mouthful, but here is the key: If you want to thrive, focusing on brain health has to be a constant condition, not one you employ every now and then. Consistency and vigilance line every path to optimum function. It happens by amplifying and maximizing what is already there and using the activities that support your life to raise the quality of your health and increase your ability to thrive. You don't have to give up anything or add more activities into your day.

That is certainly not a standard protocol in our country's healthcare mentality. When someone is *injured* in our society, we find treatments to fix their deficits.

There was a point in my recovery process where I made a shift in focus and I am not even sure I know where or when that happened. That shift moved me from seeking treatment and looking for intervention to make me better to reaching for those things that empowered me and turned up the volume on the quality of my life at that moment. It must have been one moment in time, and I imagine it was significant. Too bad no one who might remember such things was living in my head at that point.

My path to Okay was filled with a resolve to find ways to build up the good things that were left in my life. I set out to simply amplify and turn up the noise on those things I love and find ways to work through the discomfort by building quality in my life through that process.

There was a point when I realized that my body rewarded me every moment that I felt good, so why not try to repeat that? I tried to use all those activities that we know are good for our brains and turn them into things that make my experience on Earth a better one.

Here is one of my favorite examples. I love music so I find every way possible to use it as a tool. I studied the healing properties of music—brain activity associated with specific rhythms or styles or levels of complexity—and then took the experience associated with music up as many notches as my brain would handle. I worked music into so many moments in the day but, most significantly, into things that might not be so exciting (like exercise), keeping the focus on the element I love—the music. After a while, the two things became paired to me. That pairing became a new experience, one that created a feel-good experience and one I wanted to repeat. I also wanted to mix similar experiences I love into my day-to-day activities just to see what would happen.

My approach is to intentionally maximize the everyday and the routine, turn up the noise on quality, and tune in to how that makes me feel. That is not the typical health experience, but it is one that I can tell you from personal experience can make every life better. There is no subscription, no membership fee, no co-pay. You need only make a commitment to feel more and better.

Ultimately, this book is not only about brain injury or the aging brain. It is about taking what is right in front of you and using it to build a better nourished brain and a better life for yourself.

Why this book and why now?

A whole generation closely follows the aging process these days. We watch and listen as our peers and our elders lose their keys, their words, and their grasp on the connection between names and faces. We feel those things creeping into our own lives bit by bit. We want to feel in control of how we think, act, and feel. We don't want to lose our grip on the moments. We want to be able to use those moments to be, do, and think better.

There are books out there that talk about all of this conceptually and scratch the surface of how our brains age. Volumes address brain structure and function on a deeply scientific, anatomical, and research-based level. It feels like we are swimming in a sea of information that is either so simplified that it doesn't feel useful or credible or is layered so much scientific jargon and research that most of us glaze over. And then there is a wonderful but small selection of writings that dig just deep enough for us to care but rarely leave us with actionable tasks that we can fit into our already overstuffed lives.

The self-help shelves are lined with memoirs written by people, great and small, who have lived through some kind of assault on their brains, something that left them feeling the fog close in. Every single one is relevant and every single one was not only a critical piece of that individual's recovery but also a light bulb for somebody else. Books like these help people like me get through that murky, tough part of moving forward. They lead you to understand that today is the right day to start and that this moment is the first moment of the re-covery process.

Each book serves a greater purpose, diving into the particular is-sues related to specific conditions. Each helps those who need it feel that they are not fighting a unique battle and that someone got through it successfully enough to write about it.

No doubt this perspective is hugely important, but because it is usually so specific to an event-related condition or situation, it does not offer a bigger picture—one that applies across the board, including the gradual changes that come with aging.

The goal of this book is to marry what you know intuitively and what you experience every day, not just with research and useful facts but also with a deeper understanding of how your body works and how you can help it work to your advantage. The emphasis is on things you can control or guide, such as perspective, choice, and attitude. It is all about identifying a specific issue, understanding the *what* and the *why* of it, and learning how to maximize your life with practical ways to fit those actions into your day.

This book is intended to apply to a broad spectrum of brain conditions, ranging from sudden blows to the head to age-related changes, and provide information about which we know enough, right now, to act in order to make thinking and functioning better.

Nothing will work unless you do.

—Maya Angelou

CHAPTER 1

How I Got Here: My Story

I remember the sound of breaking glass. I remember reaching down and wondering why my glasses were sitting in the street, outside my car. I remember pulling my cell phone out of the pocket of my hooded sweatshirt, hearing my husband on the other end of the line, and telling him that I thought I was in an accident and was not sure the car was driveable.

I remember hearing a policeman ask someone to note that I refused to go the hospital by ambulance—thinking that maybe that was a bad idea.

I am haunted by the piercing sound of that siren. I can see my husband pushing aside the curtain in the emergency room as I sat on a cold, metal table with my arm in a sling, grasping for something that felt real.

I remember the horrified look on my husband's face as he walked away from the computer after reading my summary of the accident—the one our lawyer asked me to write so he could fill in the time gaps in the police report after I'd had a hard time telling him the story. I wrote for a living, and he and my husband knew that words often flowed more freely and clearly when I wrote them down—especially things that felt raw.

I remember feeling like the tears were burning trails down my cheeks as I realized something was really wrong, something I could not easily change or understand—even when I tried hard to focus. My words made no sense. My sentences had no structure. I jumped from thought to thought without logic or continuity. There were huge holes in the timeline and no clear details within the sequence of events.

I remember telling my husband that it was the pain medicine messing with my head and that's why I could not communicate clearly. Yes, the pain medicine created this fog and soon it would lift. I just needed some rest.

And then my husband told me I had refused to take any pain medicine because I was afraid it would mess with my thoughts and make it difficult to think. I kept grabbing for something, anything that felt solid. But every time I reached out, I came up with nothing that made any sense.

Days passed. My shins were bruised and bleeding from running into things, and my hands, elbows, and knees were full of scrapes from falling. I couldn't judge where anything was. I didn't know the coffee table—the one that had been in the same spot in my living room for ten years—was right in front of me until my shin slammed into it. Nor could I judge where the last stair was until I stepped for the landing only to find I was already there.

No balance. No depth perception. No sense of direction. No way to focus or hold a thought long enough to understand it. I was living my life stuck in a paper bag and working so hard to find the opening.

Just when I was pretty sure I was about to crawl out, it felt as though someone resealed the opening tightly and gave it a shake just for good measure.

I couldn't manage much and those things I tried to manage didn't go all that well. It took me four hours to go to the grocery store, weaving my way up and down the aisles, never really sure why I was there or what I needed. Even when I remembered to make and take a list, I followed it one item at a time no matter where each was located in the store, sometimes backtracking through the whole store five or six times. I knew I was at the grocery store, though, and that, itself meant progress.

I remember the undeniably defeated feeling that swept over me one day when I opened the freezer to put away five enchilada meals (they were five for $4 that week) and found 15 enchilada meals neatly stacked on the shelf. I'd just plain forgotten the freezer was already full because they were "such a good deal" yesterday and the day before.

I had been working for a dynamic public relations agency at that time. My days were filled with meaningful work, responsibility, and pride. But my whole world shifted the day I left the parking lot after picking up grapefruit and a loaf of bread on my lunch hour.

A woman in a minivan with two children strapped in their car seats ran the red light, slammed into the side of my car, and pushed me into oncoming traffic. The multiple impacts caused what they call a coup-countercoup injury. In plain English, my brain played pinball inside my skull as my head pivoted back and forth on my brain stem, banging into my skull—first the left side, then the right side, with equal force.

I was told there wasn't a single shard of glass left in any pane of my car; the impact and my head took care of it all. I remember the piles of shattered tempered glass on my lap, at my feet, in the street, everywhere. I think that memory has stuck because it was the only way I could process the enormity of the accident.

From what we could put together, based on the time it took for the emergency vehicles to get there as listed on the police report and what happened at the time of my phone call just as they showed up, I lost, and never recovered, at least three-and-a-half minutes. That, in brain terms, is pretty significant. Some bits and pieces came back later on, but nothing about those first three-and-a-half-plus minutes.

Brain injuries are strange things and often don't act in predictable or even visible ways. Apparently, I held it together on the scene, so much so that no one even thought to check my brain. For weeks, not a soul understood the extent of my injuries. No one at the scene, at the emergency room, and certainly not at my local medical facility looked past the fact that I had walked away from an accident which turned my car into an hourglass, with only a big fat bump on the side of my head, lots of bruising on my arm and hip, and some really stiff muscles. No broken bones. No bleeding.

"Whiplash," they said. "Give it a few days and go to physical therapy. It will pass."

I knew my local doctor well. Several years before, we had worked together to start and fund a nonprofit, school-based health clinic. He knew I was smart and tough, so he didn't dig any deeper.

What was really strange to me at the time was that he seemed more frustrated about me not answering a question he asked than figuring out that I had no idea what he was saying. That memory, like most during that eighteen-month rebuilding period, is pretty fuzzy. In fact, I might be remembering it wrong because I often don't know if what I am telling is what I really remember, what I was told, or what I filled in from vague feelings.

I do remember, though, how things made me feel, especially when it came to people and their reactions to me. That doctor, that man who knew me, missed a huge clue to what was wrong with me and could have saved me months of confusion. I know how that makes me feel now.

In the beginning, I think the real problem was that I didn't know how to tell anyone that something was seriously wrong. I was struggling to figure out what was real and what wasn't, but I was also unable to find the right words to explain what I felt. So I simply did not talk.

"Depression," they said. "It will pass." I knew I was not depressed. I knew why I was quiet; I just didn't have the words to let anyone know. I was the one who held things together, the smart one, the one who was always there with a solution. Now I had pretty much nothing and knowing that mortified me.

I guess that was the first sign that my personality and my approach to life were going to have to change in very fundamental ways if I was going to survive, no less recover.

If only I had the brainpower to figure it out.

I remember the day our lawyer, in the middle of what I thought was a conversation about getting the insurance company to replace my car, looked at my husband and handed him a business card. "Ruth has a brain injury and it is going to be a long road back," he said. "This doctor can help."

Our lawyer set up the first appointment with a physical medicine doctor—the woman who walked with me, guided me, and helped me figure out that when I knocked the window out with my head, I lost pieces of *me*. I had to find a way to be *Okay* with that.

I know how lucky I am, and I am grateful every single day. My road to *Okay* has been lined with people whose encouragement did not waver, not once, ever. I've had so much support that many others in my position do not, starting, ending with and flanked by my husband and teenage son.

I had a supportive medical team that listened, reacted, and made changes based on what I said. For the most part, they looked beyond the fact that I seemed *normal*, and they really heard me when I told them I was not happy with how I was thinking, feeling, or getting through my day. They helped me figure out *compensatory strategies* to organize my life so that every moment of every day did not feel so overwhelming. They helped me understand that hitting my head had knocked every drop of cognitive reserve I'd built up over the years out of me.

At the end of the day—and sometimes in the middle—I hit the wall, usually at full speed, and just couldn't think one more thought. There was nothing to do but accept that as fact.

So I had to get to the point where I realized it was not only *Okay* to sit and stare at the wall but that that was my way of restoring. That staring at nothing and watching *The Fugitive* or *U.S. Marshalls* over and over and over actually helped me recover from the daily head-on collisions with the metaphorical wall. Yes, *The Fugitive* and *U.S. Marshalls*. They were familiar, and even though I didn't remember the plot or any particulars about the characters, it was comforting to recognize something and not have to figure out why or what to do with it. By about week six, Tommy Lee Jones was solidly part of my support team, and I appreciated that he kept showing up to help.

Looking back, I am not entirely sure why those two movies played so often, but I certainly needed them and am grateful that they did. I remember my husband and son, at different times, walking into the room and smiling when they saw I was glued to the chase through the cemetery or the rush through the swamp because they knew I was, at least for that moment, not struggling with anything. I really should send Tommy Lee Jones a thank-you note.

My doctor/savior sent me to another critical part of my recovery team—a compassionate neuropsychologist. He understood that I was focused like a laser beam on recovery and the road that would lead me out of the paper bag I had been living in for the past month. He got it that I was frustrated and driven enough to do the work needed to rebuild. So the testing, evaluating, planning, and daily brain work began.

In the grand scheme of things, I got to that point very quickly. It takes most people many months and sometimes years to get the right kind of help. Some never get adequate support, a fact that breaks my heart. My team, one that empowered me, was in place, and I was insanely motivated to recover and rebuild.

I benefited greatly from therapies—cranial sacral therapy, acupuncture, behavioral optometry—but the real changes only happened when I pushed myself. My cognitive rehabilitation specialists gave me exercises such as reading out loud and endless paper-and-pencil challenges to spur activity in those areas of my brain that had shut down.

There is an interesting yet sobering little-known fact about the aftermath of a blow to the head. A brain injury caused by impact starts a progression of neuron death that *cascades.* One neuron dies, shutting off activity that feeds two more, so then they die. That forces a chain reaction which keeps going until it runs out of momentum or the pathways are reactivated. This cascading is not predictable nor is it preventable, primarily because the process starts and usually ends before anyone is aware that anything is happening at all.

You would think that kind of thing would show up on a scan. Because it occurs on the cellular level, though, the only way to figure out what happened and the path of cascading is to watch for changes in behavior, thinking process, emotional control, reaction to sensory information and people, and problem solving. Watch very closely. Right now, there is no readily available technology to detect cascading. Behavior change is the key, and that means someone needs to be paying attention.

My road to *Okay* was sprinkled with events—things that were significant enough for me to lock into my memory. The fact that I could remember very specific moments or pieces of conversations while the rest of my life just fell away as quickly as it happened frustrated me no end.

I discovered a funny thing about memory: The deeper the emotional value I gave a piece of information, the more likely I was to remember it. That strategy has a huge downside, though, especially for someone with nothing stored up in a reserve tank. The more I used this strategy, the quicker I depleted both my thinking and emotional power. I learned to do this very sparingly and replace it with other, less taxing (and less efficient) memory tools.

I was hypersensitive to sounds, smells, and often light. I got nervous when there were people behind me and was not at ease in public unless I was physically in a spot where no one could possibly come up behind me. Part of that was about controlling my environment. Because there was so little I could control, I fiercely hung on to those things that allowed me to feel in control.

I was uncomfortable talking to people—especially those who knew me before my accident. I looked so *normal* to the rest of the world, but the fact that nothing was normal and I had no idea of what normal was any more made me ill at ease outside my house. Those were tough things to work through.

My son was a junior in high school at the time of the accident. He was involved in sports, academic teams, and had just gotten his driver's license. I had always been involved in every community and school project and was a member of just about every steering/advisory committee. I was one of *those* people who did everything and was asked to be very public about it all. When I walked into a room, my reputation (however that was perceived) walked in with me.

What a conflict. After the accident, I frequently walked into events with a cell phone plastered to my ear pretending to be talking to someone until I found a safe spot in the bleachers, at the back of the room, or in the corner of the restaurant. Most of the time, there was no one on the other end; it was just a crutch to get me to safety without having to engage in any meaningful contact.

I lost some friends—those who just did not know how to deal with the changed me or who misinterpreted my discomfort living in the world as a change in attitude toward them. I got great support from others—a group that came over to play games with me and help me laugh at my daily quest to find my keys, my shoes, and my wallet. These were my trusted friends who made sure when we went out in public I was sitting in the corner of the restaurant or at the top of the bleachers with my back to the wall and that no one penetrated my safe zone and made me uncomfortable.

There are events that serve as pivot points in any process. Those I experienced in my foggy days were pivot points not just because they were changes in how I saw things, but also because they were big enough, emotionally connected enough, significant enough to stick with me.

For example, I remember sitting with my husband on the third floor of The Tattered Cover in Denver surrounded by books about brain injury. I picked one up and, in that moment, realized that some-one got the fact that since the accident I was so different and life so foreign that sometimes I was not sure I could think my way through the muck – she lived it, she wrote about it, and I held the proof of that in my hand. The book confirmed that I was not the only one who forgot to put water in the pot when making noodles or turn the stove off after cooking. I wasn't alone in neglecting to sign the bottom of the form so our insurance wasn't cancelled or forgetting the order in which laundry needs to be done. It validated that when I knocked the glass out of the window with my head, something life altering happened below the surface where no one could see it, and I did not have the skill set to describe it. I could finally stop trying to find the right words because they were right there, in black and white.

Here's another pivot point: I was sitting with someone in a therapy office of some kind and we were talking about my frustration at not being able to move past something. The road to *Okay* with a brain in-jury is peppered with all kinds of plateaus, and it is frustrating when all the hard work doesn't lead to improvement. This therapist, not a part of my regular team, looked at me and in what I heard as a condescending tone said something like, "I don't know why you are so unhappy. You are smarter now than most people will ever be."

Excuse me? Did she ask me to settle for so much less and be happy about it?

Oh, I was angry and defiant and determined. I stormed out of her office and, without slowing down, walked directly and literally into the wall, face first, just outside the door.

More tears, more frustration, less light at the end of the tunnel because of yet another blow to my head. Plus, I was still insulted, still angry. I found my car in the spot I parked in every time I went to rehab, closed the door, and shook with anger over the indignity of it all.

On the way home, anger turned into an epiphany. I realized we all, myself included, thought it was okay to talk down to someone who, at that moment isn't firing on all cylinders. That is, after all, how we speak to *old people* and *sick people*—as though they are children and unable to fully understand. I also realized that the only way to change this was to do something, to move forward to a point where I could help somehow. I had to take some kind of action but first had to get past that wall just outside the door because throwing myself into it at full speed was not the answer.

That epiphany and the accompanying resolve made it through my brain fog and stuck. So when my rehabilitation specialist suggested I take a class to practice some new skills, I decided to get my master's degree and focus on helping return dignity to the healing process. Yes, I know she was telling me to take a cooking class or an art history class or something like that. But I needed to push further and harder if I was going to use my experience to help others.

Based on what I learned and what I did, I started on a path to rebuild my brain. Along the way, I learned some pretty key things.

Faith is taking the first step even when you don't see the whole staircase.

—Martin Luther King, Jr.

CHAPTER TWO

How to Make This Book Work for You

To make it easy to follow, each chapter is split into sections. The first section is a conversation—an exploration of logic, intuition, and personal experience.

The second section digs a bit deeper to help you understand the science behind the topic and what is happening in your body. The goal is to realize what's going on and the implications this information can have on your life.

A third element, "Insights With Brain Injury", pops up throughout the book. These snippets show how each topic is relevant from inside the fog of a brain injury, putting the details in perspective and reinforcing the need to build up a reserve.

This is intended to help you look at how you, as an individual, process information and get through your day while considering what it might feel like when something goes wrong. In some cases, though, you will get a deeper understanding of brain dysfunction by listening to people I met along the way who faced different challenges—those presented by multiple sclerosis (MS), chemo-brain, anesthesia fog, or stroke.

You may even recognize some of these things in yourself. Brain changes are brain changes and, as I've pointed out, it does not matter if they are a result of a blow to the head or conditions related to stress or even aging. We all, at one time in our lives, face a change in brain function. Building a deeper understanding by seeing challenges through a different lens might make you more compassionate with others and yourself.

The final section of the book provides a variety of activities you can start doing right now to amplify and maximize your brain's potential. There are life swaps—everyday activity replacements or enhancements that help you take what you are already doing up a notch.

There are fit-in-your-life exercises you can add to your daily routine—short bites of activity that take less than three minutes and, again, will help maximize and even expand your brain's potential. The more intense activities can help you change your focus and elevate those elements of things you already love but don't seem to have time for by giving you another, more scientific, reason to do them.

You also will find bonuses for brain geeks—resources that help you dive even deeper into both the research supporting what you are reading and the implications for future understanding. Warning: You might find yourself fueled by a passion to learn "just one more thing," which might lead you to a whole new level.

Peppered throughout the book are discussions about topics or conditions on a deeper or more practical level. These are tools you will carry with you and can use to look at your life through a brain health-focused filter to help you identify life enhancements in your daily routine.

The Benefits of Recapping What Think We Know

We assume we are living in a world of shared experience that we see things in the same way as our neighbors and we all get the same lessons from everyday situations. The truth is, that is rarely the case. Looking at issues and conditions through a different lens helps you gain a new level of clarity and increases your chances of having those *AHa!* moments that might change your perspective.

It is important to drop those assumptions and explore other points of view. This will allow you to mix things up in your life a bit and make sure your brain doesn't get too comfortable with the familiar and comfortable patterns or maps that dictate your actions. Discussion can fuel desire to try a different approach.

Talking about what we know can open up new ways of looking at life because it uses other processes in the brain. It sends a signal to its inner workings that there is more than one path to take in virtually any situation. When you change how you look at your world, you let your brain know there are other ways to solve a problem, to create, to communicate, to explore, and to tap into experience. If, for whatever reason, a neural pathway is not available to help you think through a tricky spot or solve a problem, your brain knows it can take a different path. It has already practiced that skill when you changed the lens that you normally use to view the world.

Talking about those intuitive ideas gives you that perspective and offers your brain a distinct advantage. We will try to look at every topic in this book through a new, multidimensional lens.

Scientific Basis

Brain science can be intimidating if you try and take on too much at once. It is, however, quite useful and can even be perspective-changing to understand what is happening in your body in general and your brain in particular. That understanding allows you to see how everyday actions can help you alter the quality of your thinking. Those everyday actions are often small and, without this knowledge of how the body works, might feel pretty insignificant. When you focus on the biological roots of your thinking, you might even develop ways to regulate your internal reactions—how quickly your heart beats, the tempo of your breathing, the flow of chemicals in your body.

With that in mind, each topic in this book will be explained using a biological lens and will be presented in digestible, implementable bites that you can use to better understand how your behavior, your actions, your choices, and your lifestyle can change the way your body works.

When it comes to the body, a few basic elements are the building blocks for everything else. To be very clear, this is in no way intended to be a textbook on the brain or brain function. We will only scratch the surface of the body's complicated system of message and action-reaction and will move out of the field of traditional hard science for a few solid reasons.

First, when it comes to understanding how everyday actions can change the brain, the well of information from hard science is simply not that deep. Brain function has only been looked at intensively through the wellness lens for about 15 years. That is too short a period of time to collect enough long-term data or compile a large enough body of knowledge to build a strong library to serve as a foundation for intervention creation.

Next, people are different. Situations vary. Conditions change. It is difficult to model everyday life and replicate it in the laboratory. Behavioral brain science has to come up with a way to either control enough variables or successfully loosen the definitions sufficiently to convince the rest of the world there are some "knowns" out there and that we can apply them.

The aging brain is the next part of the mystery. Researchers have been studying changes in the aging brain for only a couple of decades. The vast majority of the initial work was done using sick or fragile subjects, where decline was not a huge surprise. So there simply has not been enough time to figure out the details of what we are facing.

We do have some evidence that leads in one direction or another, but the field of study is too new and the parameters too undefined to be widely accepted as clear cut or definitive.

In addition, the focus of research in most scientific endeavors has only recently moved to study with the intent of using the results. Think about this: Historically, scientific research was done in the name of exploring and furthering knowledge—basically doing research to spur ideas, great thinking, and new areas of study. Even in medical research, academics have frowned upon commercial use of results—almost as though it tainted the results to turn them into interventions. This was absolutely the case in studying how the brain works until very recently.

Finally, research with *soft* interventions like lifestyle changes, brain exercise, and nutrition are very difficult to study. Critics talk about how nothing can be proven because it is almost impossible to control all the variables, at least in a humane way. One set of critics says it is impossible to generalize from animal studies to humans even when brain structures are extremely similar. Others say that it is only possible to show improvements on unique tasks—those specifically used as part of the training experience. They assert there can be no linking of gains to other areas because there is no way to prove what happened in the laboratory was the one thing that made the difference.

Some call ignoring those critics "pop" science, but in many cases, that is exactly what I intend to do—ignore those critics. Not because I believe their arguments to be flawed. They are not. But is the time when it is wisest to take what we know and use it to maximize our lives even before all the evidence is in—especially when there is no downside.

I believe that time is now. If we are talking about everyday brain health promotion, it makes sense to me to take what we do know and frame it in the context of how we know the body works. Intuitive information helps when looking at applying principles that have not been thoroughly studied as long as it is put in the proper context and within the right framework. Our context is daily life, and our framework is the body.

Every exercise and suggestion in this book comes from that perspective. Use those pieces of information to live better and more fully, and know that you are working from foundational knowledge and principles. The intent is to think better and build up a reserve to draw on when things don't go exactly as planned. Start now.

With that in mind, the following is a basic brain primer and not intended to be complete or exhaustive. It will lead you through what we do know and how you can use that information to amplify your experiences and fire up activity in the brain to be good, bad, or inconsequential.

You will also need a tool kit, which you can assemble now as your first step toward healing. This kit will contain the things you will need to apply my suggestions as we follow the path laid out in this book. Here we go:

Items for Your Toolbox

- A pair of comfortable shoes
- Several pairs of shoes to change into
- A stopwatch/timer
- Access to a place to get some exercise
  - Gym membership
  - Recreation center
  - Exercise equipment
- A device that plays audio files
- Paper and pencil puzzle books, newspaper, or magazines that have things like:
  - Mazes
  - Crosswords
  - Jumbles
  - Crytpograms
  - Word searches
  - Sudoku
  - Logic puzzles
  - Photo puzzles
- Board games (and someone to play them with)
- Access to YouTube on a connected device (computer, tablet, phone, reader)
- A device to load some Apps
- A library card
- A Thesaurus
- Laundry to fold
- Something to write with
- At least one new notebook
- Something to read like
  - Books

25

- Magazines
- Newspapers
- Access to other people (friends or relatives) and online communities
- Cloth to cover your eyes (a blind fold)
- Maps

Set a deadline of one week to get your kit in order. Try to collect at least three items on the list each day. Once you've got your kit assembled, we can begin our journey together.

CHAPTER THREE

Being Self-Aware: How Your Brain Works

Your brain has two kinds of cells: neurons (gray matter) and glial cells (white matter). Neurons relay electrical and chemical messages to and from the rest of the body. These messages direct your activity and process all the information that goes in and out of your brain and your body.

Neurons, however, make up only about 40 percent of the brain. Glial cells, make up the rest of your brain's mass. These cells form a fatty layer that insulates and protects crucial parts of the neuron. This fatty coating called myelin, protects, nourishes, and regulates how your gray matter works. Glial cells are 70-80 percent fat—yes, being a fat head is a good thing if your goal is to protect your brain cells! The rest is protein, which I will describe in a bit.

Neurons must work together to create any kind of action. Alone, they are just a galaxy of cells with no purpose. But together they direct almost every system in the body. When stimulated—like when a piece of sensory data comes in—neurons use electrical signals to relay information from one part of the cell to another. That information relay takes place at a synapse—the brain's version of passing a message or action on to the next level. At the synapse, the brain then converts that electrical signal to a chemical signal in order to pass the information to another neuron. The neuron must create a chemical—a neurotransmitter—to successfully send a message in a form that can be understood by another neuron.

Brain Chemistry and Neurotransmitters

The whole neurotransmitter/neurochemical concept is huge and well beyond the scope of what we are trying to do here, but a surface understanding of a few neurochemicals and neurotransmitters will give you a solid foundational knowledge and help you see some of the interconnectivity, at least on the surface.

Let's look at the good stuff first. Dopamine, serotonin, and norepinephrine make up the trifecta of feel-good brain chemicals. These chemicals, along with a few others like endorphins, oxytocin, glutamate, GABA, and acetylcholine keep the brain regulating—both stimulating and inhibiting—your body's actions. Keeping healthy levels and a good balance of these brain chemicals is critical to good cognitive functioning in every area, from memory to problem solving to emotional control. These brain chemicals also help send correct, consistent messages to your muscles to keep you moving and to your body's systems to keep everything in good working order.

When in good balance and present in healthy levels, those chemicals turn the signals that help us function properly on and off at the right times.

These feel-good neurochemicals also serve as a reward system for doing those things that support thriving in the world. It is not only possible but also desirable to use this reward system as a tool to build a better quality of life.

Think about this: Every time you do something your body recognizes as building a better, healthier life, you are rewarded with a bath of good chemicals. It is similar to what behavioral psychology calls a conditioned response (i.e., Pavlov's dogs), but this is a biological response preprogrammed in your genetic code—a pretty cool self-fulfilling prophecy.

Regulating these neurochemicals has a huge upside as well. That's why there are prescription drugs that regulate them. Some antidepressant drugs, like Prozac, which increase serotonin, and some Parkinson's drugs, which balance dopamine release, have been shown to boost the rate of new neuron growth. Yes, that is right. Maintaining and controlling serotonin and dopamine levels in the brain's part of the vascular system actually nourish the brain and encourage healthy signal-sending (through the neurochemicals) along with new cell growth.

Stress Chemicals and Finding a Balance

The other set of brain chemicals, those that appear during stress, are necessary as well. From an evolutionary perspective, we needed cortisol releases to trigger our body's autonomic nervous system—the fight-or-flight mechanism—to protect us from harm and prepare us to ward off predators as we were out in the world, working to survive. Today predators, although a different variety, still exist. Being prepared is essential. It is so important to make sure this system works well, because threats come from all areas. We need our bodies to be prepared to fight or know when it is time to run like the wind.

Stress, a necessary condition for maintaining good brain health and surviving in the world, has gotten a bad rap. We do need some stress to keep us on our toes and to maintain a healthy level of those chemicals that nourish our brains. Fight-or-flight responses actually benefit us in small, controlled doses. They are what keep us from getting run over by buses, trains, and cars and help us assess and react appropriately to risks of all kinds.

Those who profess eliminating all stressors in your life just might be leading you down a rose-colored path. Eliminating stressors could result in your being unprepared and potentially involved in a bigger crisis when circumstances beyond your control pop up.

So how do you identify healthy stress reactions and know that you are prepared, electrically and chemically, to deal with stress? You never hear about it from your body when things are going well and all is working right—no signals, no signs, or indications of an issue. You just cruise along. It reminds me of this: I have been a boss most of my adult life, and I have had some really incredible people work for me over the years. I can count on one hand the number of times I heard someone from outside my company say out loud that these consistently stellar employees did a good job. Without fail, though, I heard from those on the outside when anything went wrong. Our bodies treat us the same way. No pats on the back to let you know that everything is working well or if stress reactions are ready when you need them. Rather, major problems occur and things go wrong.

The other stress reaction challenge is knowing when you are about to hit too much. Unfortunately, no warning bell sounds when you that line between healthy levels of stress and way too much.

Likewise, nothing signals you when you hit the point where the processes the body sets in motion as part of the stress reaction start to do damage. Too much stress is a real issue and can cause serious, long-term problems. Understanding the process, however, can help you regulate and keep the forces of stress in check.

The brain kicks off an intricate and hard-to-stop chain reaction to stress:

- The adrenal glands release adrenaline (epinephrine) to prepare the body to fight, sending a signal to other systems that it's time to go on high alert.
- The hypothalamus kicks in, triggering the pituitary gland to produce the stress hormone cortisol.
- Cortisol and adrenaline work together to maximize performance to put up a good fight.
- Heart rate, metabolism, blood pressure, attention, immune system, and the systems that regulate inflammation in the body all activate, while systems not critical for fighting, like digestion, turn off or dial way back.
- Cortisol binds with neurochemical receptors that send a message to the neurons to let in more calcium that protect the cells in the short-term.

The key is finding the right balance and maintaining the mix of brain chemicals that best support your life. Keep your stress levels healthy. Don't eliminate them altogether, because those chemicals play a role in thriving as well. Just maintain a healthy balance.

Neuro-Concepts

There are a few more *neuros* that will help pave the way to understanding the big concepts in the rest of this book: neuroplasticity, neurogenesis, and neurobics.

Neuroplasticity is the brain's ability to rewire, take new pathways, and change. The idea that the brain can do this is relatively new. Traditionally, scientists, researchers, and most notably, medical practitioners believed that the brain deteriorated with age and after some kind of trauma. We now know that simply is not true. This revelation spurred a ton of research and new inventions that attempted to capture the secret of the brain's self-repairing powers. Although the verdict is not yet in, there are a few things that have consistently come to light.

The most important thing to know about neuroplasticity is this: Change does not happen in a vacuum. It needs you and the rest of your body to help the process along. There is no magic behind the power to activate your brain's neuroplastic qualities. Healthy, balanced, stimulated brains grow new neurons, rewire, and reroute even after neuron loss or blocked pathways. Keep in mind the operative words here are healthy, balanced (both chemically and electrically), and stimulated— all factors within our control.

The other two *neuros* are the triggers for neuroplasticity and the key to open the process of rebuilding.

Neurogenesis is exactly what it sounds like—the creation of new neurons. The process of creation is the product of something much more fundamental: gene expression. We all come with an internal set of rules that direct how our bodies grow, repair, regenerate, and manufacture new material and cells. At the most fundamental level, our bodies operate by following the rulebook found in our specific DNA.

That rulebook is made up of genes, the units that direct action and set the rules in motion. Those genes *express* themselves by directing the body to create a functional product—one that allows our bodies to operate in a particular way.

Gene expression is not as complicated as it sounds. Think about it this way: When you express something verbally, for example, you give a form and context to a thought. Simply put, you give something that has meaning in your thoughts, meaning for others. You turn a thought into a *product* that someone else can understand. When a gene *expresses* itself, it takes the coded message from your DNA and turns it into a *product* that your body understands and knows how to process—a protein or a set of reactions that the body then uses to do something. In the case of neurogenesis, that protein (or other bi-product) directs your body to create new neurons.

As you age, you lose all kinds of cells including neurons. Your DNA does not stop sending messages to create new neurons to replace those that are lost. In fact, research is uncovering ways that you can actually encourage neurogenesis through action. There will be more on this in the next section, "Be Physically Active".

Neurogenesis sounds big and wondrous because it really is. Your body comes with a set of instructions that will allow it to repair itself. All you have to do is make sure the environment (your body) supports that set of directions. Just imagine what you can do if you learn how to create the ideal setting for neurogenesis.

Putting It All Into Action: Practical Application

The final *neuro* is neurobics and this concept takes us into everyday brain health and learning how to roll activities into your life. The term was first widely used by Lawrence Katz and Manning Rubin in their book, *Keep Your Brain Alive*. Neurobics relies on a few basic principles. Even though no hard science absolutely confirms these techniques work, there is much anecdotal evidence, much support from common knowledge, and great ties to the principles of how the brain works. An exercise or activity qualifies and is considered neurobic if it does any of the following:

1. Activates one or more of your senses in an unusual or unexpected context or combines two or more senses in a nontraditional way.

2. Engages your attention by doing something in a different way. The act of shifting attention and making you think is key.

3. Breaks a routine or life pattern so that you have to think, create, innovate, or refashion something you do every day.

Neurobics fit into your life and help turn everyday activities into brain boosters simply by adding a few twists and turns. Sometimes you can take what you already do and make it neurobic through simple swaps, making minor tweaks to your routine, or adding new elements to your day.

Sometimes you need to push a little harder, make the routine non-routine, and bump up the challenge just a bit to give your brain that neurobic push it needs.

"Being" Brain Healthy

In a nutshell, you have the resources, the means, and some big reasons to *be* brain healthy. Paying attention to small details in your life and integrating them into the bigger picture of *being* can help you live better, think better, and lead a fuller, more rewarding life.

There are ways to activate the pleasure centers, challenge your creativity, and maximize quality just by approaching life differently. Here is an introduction to what I see as the *"Be's"* of brain health:

Be active. There is no better way to nourish yourself mind, body, and soul than to take an active approach to life. Be a thinker, a doer, a creator, and a motivator. Move your body, use your mind, and think bigger.

Be social. Not only are we better together, but reaching out to other people also activates multiple areas of the brain. When you interact with others, you stimulate multiple areas of your brain so sensory, language, memory, logic and reasoning, and emotional areas all work in concert.

Be engaged. Participate in things that fire your passion and excite you. Some days, it is not enough to just be active and social.

Throw yourself in fully and participate in life by becoming a vital part of every experience.

Be purposeful. Find what drives you–those things that give you a reason to be—and work toward them. When you live more purposefully, you fill holes in your life and also contribute to something greater.

Be complicated. Combine activities and focuses. Make the most out of each moment by drawing from everything you know that helps you think and live better, and activate as much of that as possible all at once.

Man cannot discover new oceans unless he has the courage to lose sight of the shore.

—Andre Gide

CHAPTER FOUR

Being Active: How Your Body Can Help Your Brain

There is no better way to nourish yourself—mind, body, and soul—than to take an active approach to life. Be a thinker, a doer, a creator, and a motivator. Move your body, use your mind, and think bigger.

Move Your Body: Be Physically Active

One undeniable benefit of exercise is that, even in small doses, getting up and moving will make you:

- Feel better, more positive, and more optimistic

37

- Think better, gain perspective, and improve problem solving
- Have a better outlook on life.

Physical exercise nourishes your whole body. We have heard it over and over and over. Getting out of your chair and moving does more to make you healthy and happy than just about anything else you can do in a day. Let's get beyond this broken record and figure out how to use this information to make your life better.

In general, when you get your blood flowing and elevate your heart rate by moving your body, you not only increase your metabolism and burn excess energy, you also activate a whole slew of health-promoting processes in your body. At the most basic level, exercise focuses your whole being on wellness.

Exercising is, by far, the easiest and most direct way to alter your mood and outlook while boosting your ability to think through a problem and come up with an effective solution. These are powerful benefits, ones that immediately elevate the quality of your life in unique and wide-reaching ways.

Maybe the coolest part, the one that makes physical exercise worth the effort, is this: When you get up and move, you set in motion a process that feeds off itself and makes you want to go back for more. Your body releases chemicals that make you feel good, and those chemicals trigger other brain-based events that actively protect your muscles, feed your vital organs, and elevate your mood. You can actually feel your breathing, your heartbeat, sweat cleansing your pores, and your muscles firing on command. All the parts of this amazing machine that drives every part of your life are working in harmony.

Your body systems were designed so that physical exertion feels good. When you push yourself until you get to that *feel good* point, aches and pains fade away, you smile just a bit more deeply, and your perspective changes. All that from a little physical activity.

Survival of the Most Fit?

There is an evolutionary basis for all of this. Survival for hunters and gatherers depended on being active. It served a great purpose for the body to provide a motivating reward for moving. If our ancestors had no incentive to move, they would not have survived. The harsh reality is that not only would they not have food for themselves, but also they would have become food to faster, stronger creatures! So those who did not move quickly enough did not live to pass on the genes that wire us to want to be active.

Today, thankfully, survival is no longer wrapped up in being active. Food comes to our doorstep and, in most cases, we are pretty well protected from predators. So we now have to rely on our bodies to feed us an internal incentive to get up and move—one fueled merely by the desire to be healthy and feel good.

The hard part about this is that exercise takes time, planning, motivation, and if you want the long-term benefit, commitment. Those things are all work, so our bodies must provide a real reward to keep us moving. Enter the feel-good chemicals that nourish our bodies and our brains and make exercise feel worth the effort.

What is Happening in Your Body: The Chemical and Electrical Magic of Being Physically Active

On the simplest level, exercise increases blood flow to the whole body. In particular, though, getting up and moving brings much-needed blood to the brain. Beyond that, physical exercise helps control what is happening in your brain by altering its chemistry, keeping the electrical circuitry active, and maintaining the flow of energy, both chemical and electrical.

Let's look at what happens when you exercise in manageable units and small doses.

After about 20 minutes of mild to moderate exertion, your body starts to produce increased levels of serotonin, dopamine, and norepinephrine—the *calming* brain chemicals. Those chemicals help reset your mood, your attitude, and help you release tension.

The self-fulfilling process of nourishing your brain starts pretty quickly. When you set your body in motion with the intention of renewing and restoring, you reduce the production of stress chemicals associated with fight-or-flight (cortisol) and you increase the production of chemicals that nourish and encourage increased activity (dopamine, serotonin, and norepinephrine) in those areas of the brain that regulate mood, problem solving, and emotional control. When you push just a bit harder, your body begins to release pain reducers (endorphins) and anti-inflammatory agents (interluken-1, acetylcholine). Improved mood, pain reduction, better problem solving—there really is no chemical downside to exercise.

Intuitively, chemical balance is good, especially when it helps alter behavior in a positive way. However, it goes even deeper than that. Solid evidence proves physical exercise, even at low exertion levels, can work on the cellular level and actually help rebuild and repair cells. And in cases where there is damage, it can replace those cells lost along the way.

Something to Think About

It is a good practice to do everything possible to encourage new neuron growth. Neurons die for a variety of reasons, and many of them, like other cells in the body, fade away naturally with age. That normal aging process, however, also includes natural regrowth, all part of the process of neuroplasticity. A whole host of physical conditions exist such as disease, stroke, chemotherapy, and all kinds of trauma to the head that cut off or alter healthy activity in the brain. These un-planned events—ones not included in the preprogrammed, regrowth plan—also trigger neuronal death. Other conditions that creep into daily life and don't necessarily scream *dying neurons* but cut off nour-ishment to specific brain regions and set off the cascading effect. Stress and depression act in that way. A very common yet silent side effect of both is increased neuron death. Any time you cut off the flow of chemical and electrical activity to part of the brain, neurons die.

Setting the Stage for Neurogenesis

Let's look at how some activities have been shown to change your brain's physical environment. Regular practice of yoga (three times per week) stimulates the production of GABA—a brain chemical di-rectly related to controlling chemical depression. In conjunction with other therapies, yoga can help control the damaging effects of chemi-cal depression and actually rebuild those areas that have been affected.

This happens when you restore chemical balance in your brain by reducing the production of cortisol (the evil stress chemical), boosting production of dopamine, serotonin, norepinephrine, and GABA (calm-ing chemicals) and encouraging gene expression via the production of neurotrophins (proteins that direct cell growth in the brain). You can create a climate that is right for your body to produce new cells and grow new neurons. Focus on activities that restore balance as few as three times a week, and you will stimulate neuron growth in the areas of the brain that most frequently become damaged by stress and de-pression.

Complicated physical activity—games that require both exertion and thinking—can elevate this condition and actually help you grow new cells that will improve learning. For example, from a brain region perspective, when you play tennis, your brain coordinates multiple ac-tivities at once. It must activate processes in the cerebellum (the region that controls movement), the parietal lobe (the region that facilitates balance and depth perception), the frontal lobe (impulse control and

41

selective attention), and the occipital lobe (the region that receives and understands visual information). More on this later, but just know that by adding elements to physical activity, you can target and improve specific functions with lasting, long-term benefit.

Exercise of all kinds requires using the hippocampus—the area of the brain that is thought to do most of the work regulating memory and spatial orientation. Strong evidence shows that, on a cellular level, exercise increases gene-expressed proteins called neurotrophins that could lead to brain rebuilding (neurogenesis), in general, protecting the hippocampus and delaying the onset of Alzheimer's disease, in particular.

Brain Geek Alert: Gene-Expressed Proteins

The concepts of gene-expressed proteins, in general, and neurotrophins, in particular, go beyond the scope of this book but merit introduction because they represent a new direction in research. This line of inquiry looks at how gene-expressed proteins, activated by exercise, can help promote new cell growth in specific parts of the brain—not just increase activity in the brain but actually grow new cells. That is huge!

There are two neurotrophins and one additional gene expressed protein of note:

Brain-derived neurotrophic factor (BDNF), a protein found throughout the body but primarily in the brain, is most active in the hippocampus. BDNF has been shown to spur new neuron growth. During and after exercise, the brain produces larger amounts of BDNF.

Neurotrophin-3 (NT-3), a protein that not only stimulates new neuron growth but also encourages the generation and sorting out of new synapses. Again, NT-3 production increases during and after exercise.

Interluken-6 (IL-6), a powerfully protective gene-encoded protein, acts as an inflammation-control regulator. Researchers are looking at how exercise increases IL-6 production.

Research with gene-expressed proteins is entering new areas of study—those areas that not only look at how to change body chemical and electrical activity, but also how to encourage your DNA to work for you to maximize performance.

How much is enough to make a difference?

If you are doing cardio, more intense workouts will get your chemicals flowing more quickly. And exercising more frequently will help you maintain that healthy, nourishing level of brain activity.

Fortunately, according to John Ratey, Harvard Medical School psychiatrist and author of *Spark: The Revolutionary New Science of Exercise and the Brain*, "Even 10 minutes of mild activity changes your brain." Yes, even just taking a walk. Anything that keeps your heart pumping and your blood flowing can help keep your brain fit and active, fend off memory loss, and keep skills like vocabulary retrieval working.

Canadian researchers recently looked at how energy expenditure changed cognitive functioning for elderly adults over the course of two to five years. Most of these participants did not work out in the traditional sense. They took short walks, cooked, gardened, and cleaned. The most active participants scored significantly better on tests of cognitive function than their peers who were sedentary. By the study's end, roughly 90 percent of this active group could think and remember just as well as they could when the study began. Every little bit helps!

Changes with Brain Injury

Taking on extra activity can be challenging when physical issues come along for the ride. This goes beyond injury from an accident, blows to the head, or those physical limitations that come with such diseases as stroke, dementia, Parkinson's, or MS. You first need to assess whether an activity is suitable for one's age, fitness level, and physical ability. Beyond that, you need to consider how the activity fits with the stage of your recovery or where you are on the spectrum of disease progression.

In a *normal* world, it's logical to start slowly by just going out for a stroll. But after my accident, walking in the world horrified me and made me extremely anxious. I missed steps. I ran into walls. I tripped. I stumbled. I broke toes. And I did all of this out in the world where others could see what was (or wasn't) going on in my head.

∽

Loss of depth perception and lack of attention can be common side effects for many with both focal and diffuse brain injuries, and both get in the way of physically navigating life.

The other part of the equation is feeling emotionally comfortable. Many physical activities require being out in the world with other people moving around. That may sound silly but it is very real. When your equilibrium is off and you are hypersensitive to noise and movement (as is common after a round of chemotherapy or impact concussions), it can be extremely unsettling to be in situations in which people are out of your line of sight. Finding an environment that feels safe is critical so the effects of stress or feelings of incompetence do not overshadow the benefits of exercise.

For me, the treadmill at my local gym became a lifesaver. By giving me the ability to steadily increase the pace and the angle while holding on to first a front bar then a side bar in a safe environment allowed me to challenge myself a bit and then a bit more. I needed those tiny bites of confidence I got each and every time I stepped on that machine. They made me feel in control.

I had to find ways to feed my brain with the neurochemicals it needed to stay on the road to recovery, those that come only from being physically active. The treadmill was safe; no depth perception required. There were no distractions I couldn't control. It was just me feeding my brain with healing goodness.

I could feel the difference in my thinking after just a little bit of exercise, and I could feel my confidence building, slowly but surely.

In conditions like some types of MS and strokes, with definite and sometimes progressive physical limitations, it is important to carefully assess each activity before proceeding.

A colleague deals with the limits of MS by developing and maintaining a close relationship with her body. She has learned to listen to and respect what her body tells her. That means preplanning is not always an option because when it is time to rest, she must do so. Do a little and rest, she says. Get up and do a little more. Listen to what your body tells you, and push only as much as you safely can.

Activity That Pays You Back

Fitting exercise into an already busy schedule presents all kinds of challenges. What do you give up to fit in a workout? How can you create more hours in a day that's already packed to the brim with work, family, and social activities?

The key to making exercise worth it is to make sure that the benefits to the quality of your life outweigh the costs in time, energy, and planning. Start small. Try to roll exercise into something you already do. Involve others who you want or need to spend time with, and you might just get hooked.

Life Swaps

Here are some easy life swaps that will increase your activity level without you even noticing.

Intentionally choose a parking spot farther from the entrance. Take those extra few steps.

Take public transportation so you have to walk to the stop and your final destination.

When you must go up or down a few floors, take the stairs. Vary how you go up and down the stairs, as well. Take two at a time or walk to the rhythm of a song.

Stand up while on the telephone and while in meetings. Move your feet, walk in a circle, do a dance step—whatever it takes to get your blood flowing a bit without losing concentration.

Instead of going to lunch with a friend or colleague, go for a walk together. This works even when it is cold or raining outside. Go to an indoor mall or building that you can use as your own personal track. You might even find that ideas flow just a bit more easily and you start thinking in new ways when you walk your way through a meeting or a conversation.

Get out of the house or your office and go shopping. Yes, shopping! Think about the process. You have to get there, which means walking at least a little. If you want to take the experience up a notch, vary how quickly you go up and down the aisles or from store to store.

Fit-in-Your-Life Exercises

Can't get out of the office or leave your chair? Not to worry, here are some ways to be active while sitting that won't take away your attention or focus. Start out slowly and gradually push yourself to do more.

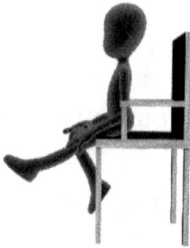

Straighten your knee and hold your leg out in front of you. Count to ten, lower your leg. Then switch legs. Alternate legs for ten times. Do this three times a day and you might really feel a difference in your thinking.

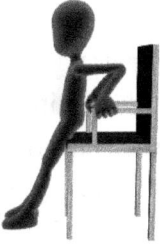

Put your hands firmly on the arms of your chair or, if your chair has no arms, place your hands firmly next to you, palms down and flat. Push down on your hands and try to lift yourself off your seat. For a really intense activity boost to your day, do five of these once an hour.

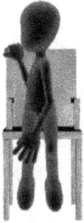

When you have a moment to look away from your screen, sit tall in your chair and stretch your arms to the ceiling. Put your left hand on your desk and grab the back of the chair with your right hand. Gently twist to the right. Hold that for about ten seconds. Let go and raise your arms, reaching toward the ceiling again. This time, your right hand goes on the desk and your left hand on the back of the chair. A couple of these really get the blood flowing.

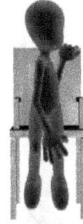

Stretches are often the best fit-in-your-day exercises.

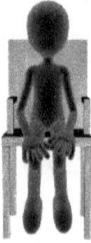

Ankle stretches: Sit in a chair with your feet hanging down not quite touching the ground. (You may also cross a leg if you need to raise your feet off the ground.) Point your toes up to the ceiling and then down to the floor. Now make a circle.

Repeat fifteen times each foot.

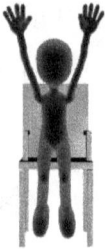

Hand stretches: Reach both hands up over your head pushing each of your fingertips as if you were trying to touch the ceiling. Feel the stretch through your hands and into your arms. Continue this stretch for 60 seconds at a time.

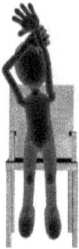

Arm and side stretches: Sitting straight up in your chair, raise both arms over your head. Grab your right wrist with your left hand and gently pull it to the left and hold for ten seconds. You should feel a stretch in your right side. Release and switch hands, stretching your left side. Repeat this five times.

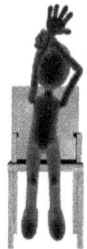

Take a yoga break with this quick routine designed to bring blood to the brain and increase energy.

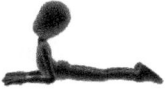

Begin with *Cobra*. Lie flat on your stomach on a soft spot on the ground (carpet, grass, sand) with your pelvic bones resting on the ground and pushing down to the earth. Extend your legs straight back behind you, with the tops of your feet square to the Earth. Your palms are flat and your fingers are in line with your shoulder blades, or if can, tuck your palms under your shoulders. Your elbows are bent and tucked into the sides of your body. As you inhale, push up from your palms, straighten your arms slightly maintaining a soft bend in the elbows as your chest lifts off the ground. Lift up only as high as is comfortable while keeping your pelvic bones and your legs pressed to the Earth. Keep your shoulder blades firm against your back. Lift through the top of your sternum but avoid pushing your ribs forward. Try to keep your back evenly curved throughout your entire spine. Your gaze is steady and looking forward toward the horizon.

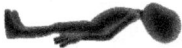

Move to *Fish*. Gently turn over to lie on your back. Arch at your pelvis and curl up your upper torso so your pelvis and upper torso are reaching up to the sky, lifting gently off the ground. Relax your head and neck and rest on the crown of your head. There should be very little pressure on the crown of your head, just a gentle stretch which should be easy on your neck. Press your shoulder blades firmly toward each other. Extend your hands overhead with steepled fingers. Your back should round slightly and you should feel a good, gentle stretch. Fix your gaze up toward the sky or to the back of room—whatever is most comfortable and allows you to achieve a gentle stretch with no pain. Ease out of this pose, gently moving your head and pelvis until you are again flat on your back with your pelvis reaching for the core of the Earth, shoulders, neck, and back relaxed.

49

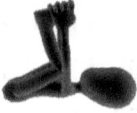

Move to *Happy Baby*. As you exhale, bend your knees into your belly. As you inhale, grip the outsides of your feet with your hands. If you can't comfortably hold your feet with your hands, use a belt or towel looped over each sole to provide some more space. Open your knees slightly wider than your torso and bring them up toward your armpits. Position each ankle directly over your knees to avoid strain. Your shins should be perpendicular to the floor. Gently flex your feet through your heels and feel a stretch through the bottom of your feet and into your ankles. Gently push your feet up into your hands (or towel). Pull your hands down toward the ground creating a bit of resistance and deepening the stretch. This should be a gentle but good stretch free from pain. Release your hands and slowly move your thighs in toward your torso and down toward the floor as you lengthen the spine, release your tail bone toward the floor, and lengthen the base of your skull away from the back of your neck.

CHAPTER FIVE

Being Mentally Active: How You Can Help Your Brain Help Itself

Thinking and being mentally active triggers many of those same pleasure centers in your brain and activates the processes that nourish your brain. It feels good to think your way through a problem or solve a puzzle. This whole thing works in much the same way and for the same reasons as being physically active. Your body rewards you for using your brain by feeding you with chemicals that make you feel good—motivation to do more and better. Positive reinforcement at its finest!

You can think about it this way. Working out your brain is a lot like working on a muscle group at the gym. You have to identify those areas that need help, find exercises that target those skills, and do the work. With any brain exercise, your goal is two-fold. You want to, first, keep those areas of the brain responsible for the skills you identify alive, active, and nourished. The second part of the goal is to encourage new cell growth in those regions and beyond.

The first part of that goal is a bit easier to zero in on than the second. For example, researchers agree that specific activities like learning new things can be directly linked to increases in both the connections in the brain (the synapses) and the chemicals that feed those connections.

⌬

Technology lets us see those connections in real time, so there is little doubt that actively thinking keeps multiple areas of your brain electrically charged and fed with neuro-chemicals. We also know, without question that when you change up a routine or add a challenge to a routine task, you can change the extent of the neural activation. Basically, you prompt activity at the synaptic connections in different parts of your brain, ones that you would not normally use to complete that task. This means you are using more of your brain to do the same thing just by changing how you approach a task. For example, if you take a walk in your neighborhood, focus on walking in a straight line putting one foot exactly in front of the other or walk on the curb. These simple changes fire activity differently than if you just walk and don't think about the process.

An active brain always builds new connections, and some research says keeping your thoughts active even promotes new cell growth. Although we don't know for sure and certainly don't understand the mechanisms yet, it is possible that using your brain inspires your DNA to create new brain cells, just like exercising your body. Enter the "Use it or lose it" approach to building a better brain!

Use It or Lose It

Use it or lose it is real in two very broad areas. First, when you use a part of your brain through active experience—thinking, focusing on sensations, picking out details, consciously paying attention to and processing the information in front of you—you fire up both chemical and electrical activity. That activity then triggers a series of reactions in the specific areas you need to use to process that information. Researchers, through the use of fMRI (functional MRI or an MRI of the brain in motion), have shown how using your brain in different ways—thinking about and even an imagining experience—actually illuminates the image of those areas of the brain needed to understand and process the experience.

Think about this: When you do a crossword puzzle, you use those areas of the brain that process language (reading and understanding the clues), association (putting the clues in context), semantic memory (providing meaning), and recall (pulling out the right word). You also use spatial recognition (fitting the word in the appropriate space, using available cues) and motor cues (holding a pen or pencil and writing). Just by keeping those parts of your brain active, you nourish them. An fMRI image of a brain actively engaged in a crossword puzzle lights up multiple areas, all of those that regulate the type of activities required.

Use it or lose it is rooted in the idea that active pathways stay alive and nourished. Dormant neural pathways eventually stop working and neurons will die. It makes sense that when you only do one thing, you ignore big chunks of your brain that need attention as well. You must, literally, use them or lose them.

Many experts agree that there is something called *cognitive reserve*—the backup that can be tapped into if something goes wrong in the brain. Cognitive reserve is that little bit of extra power saved for when the brain is under attack. Think of it as your well of support that will kick in when anything, traumatic or routine, drains all your mental energy or closes a neural pathway and leaves you completely spent.

We know that brain scientists study and provide all kinds of information about traumatic brain incidents and injuries—those that happen after an accident, a disease, a traumatic event, a chemotherapy treatment. Even though we get information about function from studying damaged brains, we also experience *routine* assaults on our brains in the course of our daily lives. Think about how you feel at the end of a tough brain day when you've worked your brain to the limits of its capacity and you are about to *hit the wall*. Or think about an emotionally taxing day that uses up every bit of your ability to think. We are talking about that *popping and fizzing* you can almost hear and feel when you reach the end of your brainpower. Your cognitive reserve is that little bit of extra brain you can draw on to soften the blow.

One leading thinker in the field and the premier voice promoting brain health is Dr. Paul Nussebaum, president and founder, Brain Health Center, Inc. and clinical neuropsychologist, adjunct professor of neurological surgery, University of Pittsburgh School of Medicine. He is shifting thinking just slightly on this issue by talking about *cognitive resilience* instead. Although the idea is similar to cognitive reserve, cognitive resilience is more about building up strength and fortifying your brain as a protective, health-promoting measure.

Dr. Nussbaum is right. The time has come to start looking at how we think about our brains in terms of promoting health, vitality, and resilience. Actively thinking, dealing with novel things or old things in a novel way, and challenging yourself, all help create paths to cognitive resilience.

The brain is amazing. It will try to use all available pathways to process information before tapping into reserves. The best way to keep our cognitive well full and available for any unplanned or uncontrolled events is to keep working to make new neural connections and create more pathways to process the world.

In other words, be mentally active. Play games, read, create, sing, learn new things. Do what makes you feel good and keeps your mind active. As long as you work to keep it full, your cognitive reserve can pull you through to a safe spot when things get rough.

Aging and Being Mentally Active

Some big changes in how we think occur as we get older. It seems that as time passes we use our brains differently. We don't use just one process to get to an answer, and we frequently get frustrated with the results when we repeat approaches that weren't quite right or that left us unsatisfied. Instead, we use more processes and, therefore, more of our brains to solve problems, access memories, and communicate most effectively. It seems like as we age, our quest for better and more extends beyond creature comforts to the quality of our thinking.

Here is a tangible example. I frequently have no idea where I put my shoes when I came home and therefore spend way too much time and energy looking for them. Yet I pride myself on my ability to not just tackle new things but also to excel and master tasks that my 20-something-year-old brain would not have considered taking on. The things I consider on my own with no help other than the research libraries I have at my fingertips—Google, YouTube, or howstuffworks.com—are a bit staggering. I had no idea how to write or format a book, but here I am writing in a format that research told me would be the easiest for working with publishers.

My 20-something-year-old self would be in awe of my ability to use technology to market, communicate, and spread the message of brain-healthy living. My 20-something-year-old self would not have been able to think and sort information much like an entire company. I am my own IT, personnel, marketing, sales, content production, and research and development departments—systematically eliminating the obstacles blocking my path as each comes up.

It just would not have been possible to imagine the breadth and depth of what I can handle now. I can do that because I have trained my brain to look for other options. I constantly challenge myself to think harder and dig deeper instead of asking for help. Given the time, I can find my way out of just about any situation.

Use It or Lose It Life Benefits

Thinking harder makes you feel better. The sense of pride that comes with solving a big problem or tackling a new task often makes the effort worth it.

When you think harder, you achieve more. Putting out the extra brainpower to get what you want and need all on your own makes the accomplishment feel so much sweeter.

Be Mentally Active: Basic Science

Thinking more actively fuels communication between neurons. In order to do something, your neurons need to work together. That means passing messages between them, using neurotransmitters and electrical activity. The process of working together keeps your neural pathways open and alive by feeding them with chemical and electrical activity. An active pathway is one that you can call on and use. The bottom line is this: You can't access an inactive neural pathway, so keeping chemical and electrical activity firing will ensure that specific neural pathway stays open. And that is critical to thinking better.

Brain Geek Alert

Researchers are starting to take a more in-depth look at cognitive reserve or resilience and how it works in the progression of dementia associated with Alzheimer's disease. There is mounting evidence that people who stay the most intellectually stimulated, are more educated, and are lifelong learners delay the clinical symptoms of Alzheimer's. On the other side of that coin, a growing group of studies seem to indicate that older people with less education, lower occupational status, and fewer intellectually stimulating activities will more likely develop the clinical symptoms of Alzheimer's disease than their counterparts. There is some hopeful and promising research out there, though.

According to a review of recent and ongoing research done by the National Institute of Health (NIH), it's still unclear which factor plays the strongest role. Does higher education itself help create cognitive reserve? Is actively using your brain the key? Are certain people simply born with more cognitive reserve and it's these people who tend to become well educated and hold higher status jobs? A few recent studies seem to point to a combination of factors.

One recent Swedish study of twins indicates that genetically endowed intellectual capacity might be the key. Another study out of the University of Southern California found that "...level of education predicted Alzheimer's disease when looking at the study population as a whole, but not when they compared twins—one of whom had dementia and one of whom was healthy—against each other." This leads to another branch of research that concludes it is intellectual involvement that provides protection from the symptoms of Alzheimer's not necessarily formal education.

Here is the summary from one prominent study out of the University of Chicago. "On enrollment in the study, the researchers asked study participants—none of whom showed signs of dementia—how often they engaged in seven simple but cognitively stimulating activities: viewing television, listening to radio, reading newspapers, reading magazines, reading books, going to museums, and playing games such as cards, checkers, crosswords or other puzzles. They found that the more cognitively active study participants were, the less likely they were to develop the symptoms of Alzheimer's disease. In fact, participants who scored in the top 10 percent on the cognitive activity scale were 47 percent less likely to develop Alzheimer's disease than people who scored in the bottom 10 percent."

This is pretty strong evidence that intellectual stimulation plays a role in delaying the onset of symptoms and supports other recent studies that take the same approach.

Unfortunately, these studies don't answer the question of why. Wilson hopes that after further data from an ongoing study of a group of nuns who have had very similar life experiences, he will find some valuable biological clues. Each nun agreed to a post-mortem brain study. To date, they have autopsy results from 90 percent of deceased participants. With those, they can start to examine whether cognitive activity reduces risk by a direct effect on Alzheimer's disease pathology or through some other mechanism such as an association with neuron numbers or synaptic density in brain regions critical for thinking and memory.

"It could be that having more neurons in a given area or more connections between the neurons makes that neuronal system less vulnerable to Alzheimer's pathology," Dr. Wilson says. "Or it could have to do with brain plasticity—the idea that some people still retain plasticity by seeking new information or manipulating new information. There are many open possibilities."

Brain Injury Insights

My brain injury made me a very rigid thinker and that, in turn, made it more difficult for me when I could not get the details just right. For example, I was not comfortable with a word that was close to what

I was trying to say. It had to be perfect. The reality was that the perfect word rarely came, and when it did, it was not easy to get there. I lost so much of the moment looking for that word that my quality of life took a serious hit.

I found it easier to focus on the task at hand and not vary outside the lines. That meant the details become more important than the process and stretching my thinking beyond the details of the moment was not a comfortable option. In many cases, being mentally active required a whole lot of skills that were not readily available: attention, focus, ability to shift and flow with a conversation, react from an appropriate emotional place, to name a few. Inside the paper bag that defined my life at that time, I had to find ways to create a safe place to think—one where I could make mistakes and not feel like it was a huge imperfection sitting there for the whole world to see.

With the help of a cognitive rehabilitation specialist and a whole lot of research, I found things that helped me get past those nagging fears. I was able to push myself, even in public, to think more and open more pathways. I spent hours every day working on skills, and that got me thinking. I tried to learn new things, and even though I did not retain much, it pushed me outside the comfortable boundaries.

Eventually, those boundaries loosened and I reopened pathways by working them. My memory improved as did my ability to cope and my confidence in my ability to think grew. There is no substitute for being mentally active. I found that *Use It and Regain It* makes every bit as much sense as *Use It or Lose It*! It is all a matter of making it fun and making it work for you.

Chemotherapy and sometimes the after effects of anesthesia can also cloud thinking and block the ability to be mentally active on a significant level. I know an extremely intelligent, highly functional young man who, for up to a year post-chemotherapy, could not re-member facts for more than a few minutes. He was taking classes—doing all the work, attending lectures, and incorporating very rigorous review techniques—but could not retain the information. He started to fail tests and lose confidence. It was critical for him to 1) speak up and let his professors know what was happening, 2) develop some *compensatory strategies*; tools and tricks to organize information so that he could find it on paper or in a document when he needed it, and 3) be kinder to himself as he got through the fog.

The key is to find a strategy that works and keep building, pushing the limits, and moving beyond.

Be Mentally Active: Life Swaps

Being mentally active in your everyday life is a whole lot easier than you might imagine. Sometimes it is as simple as mixing things up a bit or adding an element of challenge to a familiar task.

When thinking about what is happening, try to use different words to describe what you mean. For example, if you are hungry and a big fruit salad might be exactly what you need, say to yourself, "My hunger will be quenched with a colorful bowl of natural vitamins and sug-ars." Or "what I need right now is a good dose of sunshine-filled vitamin C." Reframe your thoughts and use different words.

When in line at the grocery store or in a waiting room, pick up a magazine and play word games. Take the words from the headlines and rearrange them into a new sentence. Or take one of the longer words and see how many words you can make using the letters in that word. Or, choose a color (red) and find the word that fits (find words that represent things that are red).

When going to a familiar place, take a new route. Choose an un-familiar path and reroute your mental map.

When going out for a walk, wear a different type of shoes. Try round-bottom sneakers or hiking boots or sandals instead of what you might normally choose. Changing your shoes changes your experience and helps make the simple act of getting from one place to the next more complicated by adding a bit of challenge.

At a restaurant, ditch the calculator and figure out the check, the totals, and tip in your head. Challenge yourself to practice your mathematical reasoning by using it.

Fold, hang, or put away laundry in categories. Pick out items of the same color, the same type, or the same material first. Sorting within your everyday activities is a great brain booster because it helps you shake up your routines and divert your attention to the details.

Be Mentally Active: Fit-In-Your-Life Exercises

While at your desk, choose item that you see and alternate these exercises:

Think of five different ways to describe that item. For example, a pencil could be:
- A writing instrument
- An erasable recording tool
- An eraser and graphite holder
- A No. 2 writing tool
- A sketch creator

Think of five words that begin with the last letter of the item's name that you might find on a desk. Using "pencil" again:
- Label
- Letter opener
- Laminator
- Laptop

- Library book

Identify a category that item belongs to. Name five other things that belong in that category. For example, a pencil could be categorized as a school supply.
- Notebook
- Textbook
- Backpack
- Highlighters
- Calculator

Look at the item closely. How else can it be used? Name five ways. Pencils can be used as:
- A tool to open a package
- A chopstick
- A scratching stick
- A drumstick
- A pointer

Play word games and puzzles. Some days, there is nothing like a good, old-fashioned crossword puzzle, Jumble, or cryptogram to get your brain going. Look for some nontraditional word games or those with a twist.

Do mazes. There is something so powerful that happens in your brain when you do paper-and-pencil mazes that this exercise frequently is used in brain-injury rehab. You activate multiple pathways and make in-the-moment decisions while challenging yourself to reach a goal. That combination sets off a nourishing bath of chemical activity.

Play online games and apps designed to focus on thinking processes. Search for them on the web and see what others say about them.

Read! Read silently and read out loud. Each way follows a different neural pathway and activates language in your brain in different ways.

If you have time and want to really engage mentally, take a class, research a topic, or learn a new language.

The key to being mentally active is to stretch just beyond where you are right now. Then make it novel, keep it fresh, challenge yourself, and push your limits.

Dripping water hollows out stone, not through force but through persistence.

—Ovid

CHAPTER SIX

Being Social: How Your Social Life Helps Your Brain Thrive

This is such a simple concept and so easy to do that we don't think of interacting with others as a brain-healthy activity. Being social fills great gaps and feeds your brain in highly interconnected ways while challenging you to think and react differently.

From an evolutionary perspective, humans needed groups to survive. We hunted in groups, worked in groups, relied on each other to meet daily needs, and most importantly, used the collective to survive when under attack. Our need for others is deeply rooted in survival,

65

and therefore our brains are wired to seek out those connections and affiliations.

When you look at being social in terms of modern, everyday brain functioning, an even broader picture emerges. Our brains have adapted this need for others to include not just survival, but acceptance, self-worth, and competence—all things valued in the modern world. Even beyond that, making human connections forces us to use multiple cognitive processes to understand the world and helps the brain keep those neural pathways open and firing.

❦

Not only are we wired for survival and assimilation but we also are wired to keep our brain's social pathways in use.

Be Social: Real World Benefits

Connecting with other people provides some of the most successful, rewarding, and valuable paths to happiness. Research in the field of Positive Psychology is pointing toward a great deal of evidence linking happiness to good health, longevity, and the ability to thrive. Happy people, according to this line of thinking, are more confident, more successful, and more engaged in life's issues, big and small.

It makes sense. Relationships make you *feel* more, and since everything that goes along with triggering emotions keeps the brain nourished with all those great chemical and electrical rewards, simply turning on that process works wonders.

It's hard to match the feeling you get when you are surrounded by people who lift you up. Friendships, a strong support system, and people who challenge you increase the quality of your life in ways that are difficult to measure. It is those positive interactions, those hard to define surges of confidence, and that sense of belonging that fire up the emotional and the self-esteem centers in your brain and help you find your place in the world.

You are, without a doubt, happier when you have someone to care about, with whom you can celebrate, share ideas, and be yourself. Research into happiness has produced some varied results, but the one unifying theme is that humans are social animals who are just plain happier when they're with other people.

Even though that makes total sense when exploring personal relationships, the effect is magnified when considering the benefits of belonging to groups. Groups feed off one another's emotions and build on and magnify the mood. Positive people will be even more positive when they're in the company of those with a similar focus on finding the good. A great way to change your attitude and shift your perspective is to put yourself right in the middle of a group of positive people.

These days, not all positive interactions take place face-to-face. You can easily find supportive social networks online as well. Groups that share a passion, a skill set, or a condition in life can be empowering and uplifting when approached with a good attitude and an intelligent perspective. This becomes extremely useful for those who can't get out or have issues that prevent being comfortable in a social world. Supportive social groups are perfect places to test skills, gain confidence in your ideas, and build those pieces of self-esteem needed to take life to the next level. Preaching to the choir works wonders, and the praise you get from your peers helps build a better you.

A strong cautionary note, however: There are also a host of negative groups that, if you are not careful, can pull you into a downward spiral. When looking at joining or becoming part of any kind of social group—whether it is face-to-face or online—look closely at the tone of the conversation. Are comments helpful and supportive? Do members treat each other with respect? Watch for those signs of negative undertones or criticism.

This evaluation process can also be a great brain workout. When you look at seeking social interaction as a cognitive challenge, you are, according to plan, turning an everyday activity into a brain booster. Keeping the focus on moving your emotional spiral in an upward, not downward, direction will serve you well in terms of healthy brain functioning and amplifying the quality of your life.

Really Cool Fact about Being Social

A study published in *Health Psychology* proposed this empowering conclusion:

> "People's happiness depends on the happiness
> of others with whom they are connected. This pro-
> vides further justification for seeing happiness, like
> health, as a collective phenomenon."

And from a brain health perspective, it justifies seeing being connected with others as a path to happiness. Nourishing our brain with those biologically based actions happen naturally when we are happy.

Be Social: How It Works

Just adding people to your life forces you to use brain processes that integrate and interpret information on a higher level. That is a pretty dramatic change in how your brain works and the level of activity within your brain. People add color, variety, and unpredictability to your cognitive life. Reacting to situations where all the elements constantly move, like other people's behavior, is challenging and sometimes slippery. When you are with others—whether in a social, working, or learning environment—and you figure out how to behave, you must also factor in processing other than your own and react accordingly.

❧

Bobbing and weaving your way through social interaction forces a layered and interrelated cognitive process that may take you out of your comfort zone but definitely feeds you and makes you feel good.

Think about all the different skills you need to use to fully understand what is going on:

- Attend to all the sensory information
- Pick out any threats to either self or environment
- Evaluate the position, mood, objective, and perspective of others in the conversation
- Gauge how to react, what is appropriate, and how your message will fit in the situation

Being social takes multitasking to a whole new level and requires quick thinking and reacting.

Being Social as a Way to Add Quality

Being social adds to quality of life and helps you navigate your day-to-day activities more steadily. Interacting with others forces you to activate both higher- and lower-level thinking processes. It creates a unique situation where all these processes must work together to get a full, accurate, usable, storable picture of the world at that exact moment as you live it. You use all kinds of cues with other people that you don't use when you are alone. These cues help you understand, process, and get involved with what is going on around you. When you are alone, you don't have to pay attention to body language, voice intonation, movement, expressions, and level of attention. These all add layers of information to the scene and add color and perspective to your life.

Online interaction is even more multilayered because you miss vital cues that allow you to determine the mood, tone, or authenticity of the interaction. Filling in the gaps can be tricky and you often fill in emotion or what you see as unstated content that just might not be there at all. It's important to set boundaries, speak frankly, and when in doubt, ask those with whom you communicate what they mean if the message is unclear.

Mix your reaction to others with their reactions to you and you have a wide variety of information for your brain to process. From a functional perspective, you not only use those cognitive processes that help you understand the world, but you are also add human—therefore, changeable, variable, and emotional—information to the scene. How appropriately you respond depends on how well you integrate everything in that scene. Those are big, complicated tasks that require varied thinking.

Be Social: How It Works In Practice

Below the surface of human interaction lies a set of skills that some who study psychology and human behavior call *social cognition*. This approach to looking at how we both understand the world and act proposes that behavior in the presence of others results from an internal cognitive process and not one wholly influenced by the environment. You see, process, and interpret what is going on around you based on a set of rules you developed over time and use to evaluate the world. Ultimately, you use that set of rules and its framework to determine how to act in social situations more than you use current environment or situational cues. This is called a cognitive construct and this particular construct, the one that steers social interactions, has been time-tested and shapes your behavior in social settings.

When put in perspective and applied to daily functioning, this approach makes a lot of sense. Successful social interactions involve observing and predicting other people's behaviors and responding appropriately. Think about this. When you learn from others, swap stories, laugh, and explore another's point of view, you assess motivations, emotional content, and point of view from that person's perspective. It forces you to think differently. It often feels like a synchronized dance of judging and reacting to each other's moves and a mutual adaptation to stay in rhythm. For most, this dance is not uncomfortable because we have a set of rules to guide the process. When another person's rules match your rules, the social interaction, and therefore the dance, moves smoothly and easily. When your rules don't align, social interactions become challenging and contentious.

The crux of social cognition and how it relates to everyday brain health is this: It focuses on how information is processed, stored, represented in memory, and later used to perceive and interact in a world filled with people in context. Social cognition is especially useful when considering perception, attitudes, stereotyping, prejudice, decision-making, self-concept, social influence, and intergroup dynamics.

That process of matching rules and gauging each other sets all kinds of brain processes in motion. What's truly unique about social interaction, though, is that it requires all those processes to work together in a flexible, ever-changing manner.

Be Social: The Brain Science Behind
What Happens in Isolation

Although many studies using animals look at the benefits of social interaction, at this stage in our scientific development we don't really have the ability to adequately isolate how being with other people changes us. It is nearly impossible to remove the rest of the variables that creep into life and look purely at the pluses and minuses of being social.

People are complicated creatures and our environments reflect that. With that in mind, what follows is one of those cases where we can glean valuable information by looking at what happens as a result of gross misfortune and mistreatment of humans through a retrospective lens.

After-the-fact studies of children kept in isolation for long periods of time show changes in both the structure and function of their brains. Long-term effects seem to be related to a dramatically decreased production of a protein that triggers normal, healthy brain growth and include:

- Abnormalities in the white matter, the fatty portions, of the brain. That manifests as thinner layers of fatty coating on the nerve axons. That coating, the myelin sheath, regulates communication between cells
- Interruption of normal synaptic development—the connections between neurons are lost or never established from lack of use
- In some even more extreme cases where children were subjected to gross neglect and complete sensory deprivation, the entire brain was up to 30 percent smaller

Be Social: The Pain of Loneliness

Consider the language you use to describe how it feels to be isolated. You might use such words as *pain* or *aching*. When studied in the laboratory, the reported *pain* we associate with social isolation and rejection registers in the same areas of the brain as some kinds of physical pain.

Brain Geek Alert: Taking a Closer Look at Types of Pain

Understanding how we process pain, both physical and emotional, can shed light on why isolation damages the brain and affects quality of thinking.

The pain network in the brain consists of several interconnected centers: the dorsal anterior cingulate cortex, the somatosensory cortex, the thalamus, and the preaqueductal gray. These areas each light up to varying degrees during a variety of types of reported pain. It does not matter if the pain comes from a cut, a problem in an internal organ, or an emotional condition, it still registers in those areas of the brain and is seen by the body's systems as a call to action to heal and repair. Systems react as if the body is under attack, and that triggers the appropriate chemical and electrical processes: systematically turning on protective systems (preparing to fight) and turning off routine systems (those that maintain the body's balance). The type of pain is not relevant because the reaction in the brain, chemically and electrically, is exactly the same.

The fact that the brain processes very different types of pain the same way is not that surprising to Nathan DeWall, Ph.D., a leading researcher in the field of social isolation and social pain. Using the same signaling is merely the body's way of being efficient. "Instead of creating an entirely new system to respond to socially painful events, evolution simply co-opted the system for physical pain," he says.

Dr. DeWall takes this idea a step further. The body's need to repair does not turn off on its own. If the body stays in crisis mode, long-term damage is inevitable. Dr. DeWall has been looking at ways to turn off social pain and recently published work on the effect of using acetaminophen to regulate social pain. "Given the shared overlap, it follows that if you numb people to one type of pain, it should also numb them to the other type of pain." This is an interesting angle on a highly complex problem.

Brain Injury Insights

Feeling isolated and alone was a huge issue for me after my brain injury, especially when I was out in the world working to live. That sounds odd but I was different, the world was different, and I had no idea how to react to others. I think the best way to understand this is to change perspective. Imagine this scenario: We have known each for ten years. Our children have been in the same small school, played in the same sports leagues, and taken part in the same academic events since first grade. We worked together on community projects and know each other socially. You see me in the stands at a basketball game and I look like I did last month when we had lunch. The only change is that I am on the top row, back to the corner, by myself. Maybe I had some work to do, or maybe all the seats front and center were filled when I arrived. You wave a greeting, smile, and make a comment about a book you loaned me. I give you a blank stare followed by embarrassed mumbling and an uncomfortable silence. I know who you are and how we fit together, but my brain is so busy struggling to make sense of the noises and the lights and the activity that I just don't have any processing power left to deal with one more thing, especially a really complicated thing like the dance of human interaction. It then becomes uncomfortable for everyone, making me feel even worse.

In a situation like that, the world did not feel safe to me for one simple reason. I did not have the cognitive resources to understand the scene. In the eye of a brain injury, complicated things like being social don't just overwhelm, they paralyze. Controlling the dose and the environment are keys to using this valuable brain booster as part of recovery.

I spoke with one of my colleagues with MS about the challenges of being social when her symptoms take over. Some days, when she can't feel her leg, it drags and she stumbles. Not feeling physically competent and worrying that she is being judged is socially isolating and painful. One of her best strategies for combating this is to surround herself with people who understand. People who realize she is not drunk or wounded but doing her best to get through that moment. People who realize that sometimes she needs to fill her tank along the way and rest.

Taking a Closer Look at the Social Research on Social Pain

Being social is good for your overall health, according to a meta-study which reviewed 148 other studies addressing this issues. It evaluated at the impact of the strength of social relationships on survival rates in people with potentially fatal conditions.

Overall, the rate of surviving severe conditions increased for those who had strong social relationships. In fact, they were 50 percent more likely to survive critical, acute stages of disease than those who had weaker social relationships.

Further, the strength of social relationships is just as good a predictor of survival as the longstanding, well-established behavioral measures (smoking and alcohol consumption) and a better predictor of survival than either obesity or inactivity. The studies reviewed were not all focused specifically on social relationships and survival. Other variables probably swayed the outcomes. As a result, the investigators suggested their findings most likely grossly underestimated the real impact of strong relationships on survival.

Powerful stuff. These staggering conclusions hold strong implications for how we treat people with life threatening conditions.

Digging More into the Relationship Between Being Social and Overall Health

Just how much does your brain value the time you spend with people you care about? A few facts. Spending time with friends lowers blood pressure and can reduce inflammation in the body. Those two facts just might decrease the probability of suffering a stroke or a heart attack.

Surrounding yourself with people who have healthy lifestyle habits and focus on wellness has been shown to lower stress and reduce that pull toward depression.

Because of the complicated nature of interacting with others, any social activity fires up your brain and helps fight off thinking problems. Some research claims that you can actually stabilize cognitive decline, improve mood, and elevate outlook on life when you spend time doing things with friends who are younger.

Staying socially active has been tied pretty definitively to improvements in both learning and memory. Granted, there are other factors and considerations and it is nearly impossible to control all the variables, but comparison across the lifespan between those with good social support and those without indicate this is true enough to get behind and implement.

The director of the Stanford Center on Longevity, Dr. Laura Carstensen, has been very vocal about this one point: "It's not the number, but rather the richness and depth of relationships that counts." Close connections are key.

Be Social: Life Swaps

There are so many ways to make subtle changes in activities you already do to turn them into social activities. Here are a few ideas.

Planning a trip? Try adding in some day trips with a group. Being with others just might enhance the experience. And you might come away with some new friends who share an interest or passion.

Do you take walks or go to the movies? Find a group to walk or watch with. Give meetup.com a try and link up with like-minded people while doing something you planned to do anyway.

Need to learn a new skill for job advancement or personal interest? Look for a Facebook or LinkedIn group that focuses on that area of interest. Sharing ideas and being social online while doing something you need to do will help activate your brain in novel ways and keep you challenged.

Silly as it sounds, strike up conversations with people while you wait in line. Comment on an item in a grocery basket, strike up a conversation about an outfit, or ask a question about where you are. All will help you connect and keep your brain active during those idle moments.

If you work out, try an exercise group. It doesn't matter whether it's an aerobics class, yoga, or weight training. Just move your solo workout to a group activity. You might meet people who share your interests and enjoy some new conversations.

Be Social: Roll in Your Life Activities

Oh, the things you can do every day to connect with others! The key is to connect with someone every single day.

Make a phone call. In this day of texts, Facebook messages, and online chatting, a real phone call is good for both you and the person you call. You react in the moment to what the other person says, and it presents more opportunities to really trigger some emotions.

Find something you love and find a way to make it a group activity. If you love reading, join a book club. If you love to watch sports, join a fantasy football league. If you love playing an instrument, join a local musical group. There is usually a way to turn something you love into a group activity so you can be social.

Even if you are not outgoing, push yourself to start conversations with people. Ask questions at a specialty food store. Strike up conversations with people at an event. You might even feel yourself getting more positive and confident.

CHAPTER SEVEN

Being Engaged: How to Live Your Life More Fully

Unlike any of the other sections in this book, being engaged is purely a mental activity. In this context, "Be Engaged" implies that you use internal processes to conjure up images, direct activity, and spur those systems in your body that support great brain health.

There are good reasons to limit and narrow the definition of engagement in this manner—all intended to separate what we're talking about here from other web-marketing focused interpretations of the concept. The word *engaged* has been overused and the concept of engagement overextended in current literature on web-based business

79

practices. Social media and web gurus have tried to turn engagement into the science of hooking people's attention.

In our context, be engaged means firing up those biological systems that support good health in a very efficient way. Let's look at what we mean through this simplified lens. It is quite possible to walk through each day without noticing what we're doing. We all go through periods when days come and go without being able to identify anything significant or memorable that happened. Those mechanical days just float by without fanfare, without being recorded in our easily accessible memory.

There is a big difference between living your life and being engaged in what is going on around you. Even when you are minimally engaged in your life, you create memorable events and, at the end of the day, you can identify what happened, how you felt, and what actions you took and still need to take. You thought about what was happening both in the moment and afterward. That, on the simplest level, defines being engaged in your daily life.

Now, let's dig deeper. From a brain-health perspective, being engaged in something means activating a cognitive processes. *Brain engagement* is that simple—think about, sense, recognize what is happening, and the process naturally begins. All you have to do is pay attention and acknowledge.

Thinking about a topic, item, task, feeling, plan, relationship, or whatever grabs your attention will set in motion a sequence of events that triggers a chemical release and sends messages to prompt more activity. When you pull in more sensory data beyond what you see— sounds, tastes, smells, temperature, textures—you activate and engage more brain processes and fuel more activity.

Some days it feels easier to just get through it all—to not get involved, move beyond the moment, and wait for something better to happen.

One of the great things about intentionally engaging in your life and turning up the volume on your experiences is that you really don't need to expend any extra energy—you just shift your focus. The benefits far outweigh the effort.

When you intentionally engage in your life with the idea of amplifying an experience, you will:

- Feel better physically, mentally, and emotionally
- Act more positively
- Increase the quality of the everyday
- Turn those routine tasks—the things you must do to get through the day successfully—into life enhancers

In much the same manner as when you are active or social, your body rewards you for being engaged by releasing chemicals that trigger electrical activity. This spurs action and that feels good. You can start that whole self-nourishing process just by thinking, not much extra effort required. Just think.

If the goal is to grow new brain cells, make new neural connections, and keep your brain active, engage more fully in your life.

Engage Your Senses

One easy change you can make every day will help build your brain's reserve and open up new pathways. As a bonus, this one simple shift will allow you to think about and experience the world in a fuller, richer, more engaged manner while firing up the chemical and electrical qualities that keep your brain pumping.

The one simple shift: Tune into your senses. When you see, feel, taste, hear, smell, and understand your surroundings on a much more active level, you create multilayered images and multidimensional cues. All of that will not only help you remember an event later, but will help you dive into the actual moment more fully. Amplifying an experience by adding the layers of sensory color makes your brain work harder and keeps it active and alive.

Adding more sensory data challenges you to think on more than one level and in more than one way. Information and experiences flow easily into multiple categories and have layers of meaning and associations. From your brain's mechanical perspective, that means you fire up more than one neural pathway in your brain and send the message that there are many ways to evaluate what is going on. By using more cues and adding more layers to the moment you signal that, in case of emergency (such as a pathway not working or inaccessible), your brain knows it can understand information in more than one way. How efficient to have multiple pathways, multiple ways to deal with, understand, and problem solve in the real world even when the conditions may not be ideal.

Thinking Beyond the Message

Let's try an exercise that illustrates the value of opening multiple sensory pathways in your brain.

Find a thick piece of material that fits around your head to cover your eyes and block out light. Tie that across your eyes and close them so you do not try to adapt to any visual images. Sit quietly and pay attention to everything.

At first this might be an uncomfortable feeling. Sit with it and just breathe. Does this feel awkward? What cues are there and available for you to use? Think about what you are doing to understand your world, keep yourself safe, and get through the next moments.

When you cut off your primary sense, you cut your lifeline to understanding the world. Chances are your brain will try to create mental images and use visual cues. This is a bit of a dramatic example of a pathway—interpretation through sight—being shut down, but it illustrates what happens when you lose an ability.

Just like the muscles in your body, you have to work in many directions to function at your best. Long-distance runners train specific sets of muscles to withstand the rigors of the run. Even though that runner is, by most standards, in great physical condition, his body may be sore after a mountain climb, bike ride, or a day dancing at a music festival if these are unfamiliar activities. He is using a whole different set of muscles—ones not trained to be in prime condition.

When you train your brain to try alternative routes and use other pieces of information to understand the world, you prepare yourself for a crisis. If a pathway shuts down, you can zig or zag as needed while limiting the strain and pain of doing something in an entirely different way.

Sensory Messages in the Brain

Images from research let us know that heightened sensory experiences light up multiple areas in your brain. When you bite into an apple and feel the resistance as your teeth break through the skin, hear the crunch, and taste and smell the sweet and tart flavors and aromas of the fall harvest, you are fire up activity in your brain. The process of triggering those brain regions that recognize smell, textures and temperatures, taste, and sound along with what you see bathes all those pathways with good chemical and electrical activity. Those connections keep those pathways—the direct routes to experiencing the world—open, nourished, and ready for action.

In addition, your brain synthesizes the information and makes sense out of the whole experience. That means activating some higher-level brain processes, as well. Amplifying a sensory experience creates a whole new set of information that the brain uses, well beyond the raw sensory data you started with.

Attention, Perspective, and Being Engaged in Life

At any given moment, so many bits of information buzz around us and compete for our attention. You must use what you know and what you sense as a guide to sort through the flood of information and pick out which bits of information to process, use, and store. The vast majority of the time, attention and focus are choices and must be intentional. It's up to you to decide, based on some set of criteria, what you let into your awareness right now.

Think about this: You have zero percent chance of being engaged in some part of life if you do not notice it. The reality is you can't notice everything—you have to make choices or life and a chance to dive in more deeply will pass you by.

Paying attention to the details sometimes means taking a closer look at the scene to see all the little wonders that provide information about the moment. Just remember there is great danger when you stay so focused on the small stuff that you forget to look up.

The key to taking in as much as possible is to intentionally change your perspective.

Change Your Perspective to Take In Much More

Your view on life won't change by itself—you have to make a shift. Try these minor adjustments and see what happens.

Change your "view." If you usually sit in a specific chair at the table, move to another position. If you take a designated route to get to the store or the bank, switch it up. If you change what you *see*, you change the experience and get so much more out of it.

Approach routine tasks as if you have never done them before. I remember hearing someone describe this as being a tourist in your hometown. Looking at life through a fresh lens changes your perspective. It is a great technique to use, anytime, not just when you are bored or feeling burned out. Looking at a situation as if you were seeing it for the first time can help you problem solve, recharge your creativity, or spark a renewed interest.

Seek out a differing point of view and try to dig into the how and why. When you look at an issue from the other side and really try to understand that angle, you force yourself to challenge your assumptions and put all the higher-level processing skills through the paces.

Engage In Your Life: Make Sensory Experiences Neurobic Activities

Let's go back to the criteria for a neurobic activity to see how it fits here. Engaging your senses more fully and expanding on how you see that experience hits both of the first two points:

1. Activates one or more of your senses in an unusual or unexpected context or combines two or more senses in a nontraditional way
2. Engages your attention by doing something in a different way.
    The act of shifting attention and making you think is the key.

Shifting and expanding your sensory experience absolutely qualifies here. If you add details—ones not on the surface—you create a fuller picture.

Push your experience beyond what is present in your immediate sensory world and you have this covered. Challenge yourself to create a new experience out of the everyday.

Be Mentally Engaged: A Deeper Look
at Brain-Healthy Thinking

Let's look at what happens in your body when you start a cognitive process triggered by an experience.

The easiest way to understand what happens to you when you heighten an experience is to do an exercise that takes you through the process and breaks it all down. As we go through this, keep in mind that the more deeply you dive into an experience, subject, or task, the more areas of your brain you activate, the more chemicals you release, and the more electrical activity you spark. When that is a good experience—one that is positive or challenging or complicated on a rewarding level—this activation will lead to better feelings, more excitement, and heightened enthusiasm.

There are so many ways you can take an ordinary experience up a notch by adding some simple twists and becoming more fully engaged.

Fire-Up Your Senses: Experience It

In this exercise, just use your imagination. There's no need to actually do anything beyond imagining. Follow along with this example.

Think about an everyday activity, fill in all of the details, and amplify it.

As we go through this exercise together, be acutely aware of the process your thoughts have started and how that process makes you feel. What systems in your body has the image you are about to conjure triggered?

Imagine that you are eating the most delicious thing you ever tasted. Imagine it fully. Add the layers of aromas, textures, flavors, sensations. Fill in the setting and put it in context. Include everything that made the act of eating an epic experience—all of it.

Just thinking about the topic, I started smiling and salivating. Messages raced to the muscles in my face and to the glands that signal that rush of saliva.

The best thing I ever ate was a piece of pineapple. The thought of that piece of pineapple triggered a rush of saliva and my heart fluttered just a bit. My husband and I were on one of the most beautiful, untouched trails in the world on the tiny volcanic island of Dominica. (Not the Dominican but Dominica—huge difference.) Thinking about the scene sets off a wave of calm and good thoughts. My heart rate slows, my breathing evens, my mood elevates so I know my happy chemicals—dopamine, serotonin, norepinephrine, and probably a bit of oxytocin—are flowing. As that calm takes over, I also know my stress levels are dropping. That signals my hippocampus to shut down cortisol production and send messages to all those systems necessary for good functioning that get turned off during stress (like digestion) that it is okay to run at normal levels.

We were about three hours in on our way to one of two known boiling lakes in the world. The hike had been intense and the path challenging. We studied our surroundings and noticed birds, plants, and geography we had never seen before. Bits of invigoration, anticipation, and excitement creep in as I remember the adrenaline rush that kept us moving, protected our body's systems, and helped hold off the muscle ache that we would feel as soon as that numbing rush wore off.

The great thing about merely remembering is that my system does not have to go into preservation mode and I can put the memories of the physical challenge, stamina, and endurance into a safe, nourishing place. The power of thought is completely at work here, creating a safe environment for me to get a low-impact dose of incredible chemical and electrical activity.

Our guide—a wonderful, local young man—who, no more than five minutes before pulled me up on a rock (my legs were not quite long enough to make the span on my own) took out a long knife. He lopped a pineapple off a tree, and expertly carved it into chunks. He handed each of us a piece. Its juices dripped down my arm as I took the sweetest bite of my life…. Flood of saliva, incredible sense of well-being and peace were all revisited.

I remember thinking this was as close to *perfect* as I would ever get. The sound of the wind and the birds and the rustling trees. The feel of three hours of sweat on my skin drenching my shirt, soaking through to my backpack. The anticipation of seeing something oh so rare and spectacular. And this, like no other, piece of pineapple—so sweet, fibrous, and cool—right at the center.

This memory just activated a process that took me on a brain-nourishing journey that will now last for hours. In the process, I created an environment in my body and in my brain primed for growing new cells including brain cells.

The truly great thing about getting more engaged with your life by activating your senses is that it does not have to take a lot of extra effort, be complicated, or be time-consuming. Roll more into what you already do, then revisit and reactivate later.

Science Behind Sensory Stimulation

Frequently we gain the most information about how processes work in the body by looking at what happens when things go wrong. Neuroscientists have learned so much by studying the aftereffects of brain injury.

Just a quick note on brain-injury. There are two kinds of brain injury: focal and diffuse. Focal brain come from direct blows to the head that cause a localized, specific, identifiable injury. It's helpful to study these injuries because behavioral changes can be tied to a specific area of the brain, and scientists can then make assumptions about what that area of the brain does.

More frequently, though, brain injuries are diffuse. These occur as a result of the brain banging around inside the skull after a rapid acceleration/deceleration cycle, like in an accident or fall. There is no localized center for the injury. This widespread damage frequently grows due to a cascading shutdown and cell death that goes like this: A set of cells stops working, and all the activity in that neural pathway stops. That means there's no activity or nourishment to that area and every other area down the processing line from that spot. Think about what happens when a series of dominos fall—one piece knocks down the next, which knocks down the next, and continues until nothing is left in the path. Taking away nourishment (blood flow, neurochemicals, electrical stimulation) in this kind of diffuse injury creates a cascading path of destruction because there is no nourishment or stimulation for the cells down the line. The brain needs to reroute and rewire to compensate.

Here is another really important part of that scenario. Some parts of the brain turn on activity (excitatory) and some turn off activity (inhibitory). The brain needs to know how to behave, where to send messages, and how to access the information necessary to act appropriately. Without the correct balance of turning on and off, your senses don't work well and it becomes difficult to process efficiently. Unregulated systems spell trouble. Not being able to pinpoint trouble spots compounds the issues.

We can actually learn a lot from these broader injuries. Almost all diffuse brain injuries carry with them some sensory misfires. TBI sufferers often are either overly sensitive or can't recognize specific types of sensory information. They may not respond normally to things like sounds or light or temperature on their skin. Food often tastes and feels strange, and certain smells trigger unexpected reactions. The on/off switches in the brain do not function properly and the flow of information across regions is not quite right.

Because researchers can isolate sensory data, they have been able to determine that these sensory signals are received, processed and categorized by a series of communications between specific areas and across regions of the brain. Understanding, processing, and acting on sensory data requires accessing memory, making comparisons, and using problem-solving skills and logic. From a brain-injury perspective, it means that because you use more of your brain to process sensory data, when parts of that chain of communication shut down, glitches show up in how you process that information.

Insights from Brain Injury

I had a diffuse brain injury—the result of my brain bouncing around inside my skull. By the time anyone noticed there was a problem, there was no way to accurately pinpoint the areas where the injury started and no way to identify what symptoms came first. I just knew they were all there creating anxiety and stress.

I got distracted by noises and smells and that made me very uneasy. The only way I worked through that was to "practice" living, in a nonthreatening environment—one where I could break down and it would not hurt anyone or anything. I kept pushing the boundaries of what was comfortable, introducing smells and sounds and breathing through the process, all in the safety and protection of my house.

Sensory sensitivity is a condition I muscled my way through because I needed it to go away so I could be comfortable living in my world. That drive came from a really basic need. The end result was greater, though—an opening my life to new experiences and ways to practice what I needed in a safe place.

This started a change in perspective for me as I continue my journey. I now know that I can repair, rebuild, recoup, and restore while amplifying all those things that make my life good and enjoyable. I just turn up the noise on my sensory experiences and let the rest run its course. Pretty cool, long-term, life-enhancing discovery.

Direct Your Thoughts: Be Mentally Engaged

Another less obvious way to be mentally engaged is to actively direct your thoughts. This can take many forms. The most common, though, come from a focusing or centering activity like yoga, meditation, mindfulness, or other directed or guided stress reduction or relaxation technique.

This is a pretty hot topic in research right now and there is growing evidence that directing your thoughts can help you:

- Reduce stress
- Increase focus and creativity
- Reverse memory loss
- Maximize feelings of well-being
- Decrease depression symptoms
- Boost energy
- Improve mood
- Improve quality of sleep
- Control inflammation
- Elevate outlook on life
- Create feelings of personal control

91

The key factor is this: Practice a method that allows you to direct how you think, which makes it possible for you to control chemical releases in your brain.

The more actively you participate—the more engaged your efforts—the more likely you are to feel both the short-term quality-of-life benefits and long-term brain-protective and brain-building benefits.

Recent studies have made some preliminary links between regular meditation and larger amounts of gray matter in both the hippocampus and the frontal lobe—those areas that help control emotions and focus.

Additional studies now make a connection between meditation and slowing age-related loss of gray matter in other areas that affect cognitive processing.

Several more studies reveal significant changes in density of gray matter and cortical thickening after regular mindfulness practices—increases in gray matter in the hippocampus and insula in particular.

These are all promising and hopeful findings that indicate the repeated practice of directed thoughts can actually add gray matter to your brain.

A Deeper Look at Brain Engagement

Did you know that you can engage your brain in an activity just by thinking about something? You don't actually have to do anything. Just think about doing it! Crazy concept but researchers have studied and mapped what happens in the brain when we think about an activity and compare it to the images of actually participating in that activity. Initially they were surprised that, in most cases, the images generated by a functional MRI were not that different when simply thinking about an event or activity. Actually, the more emotionally charged the thought, the more similar the images.

Be Mentally Engaged: Life Swaps

There are times during the day when you will find yourself drifting and feeling stagnant. You can actually change that by modifying your approach slightly.

The first step is paying attention. Notice how your body reacts to how you feel.

- Is your breathing even and easy?
- Is your heart regular and steady?
- Is your internal temperature even and comfortable?

You can use this information to make adjustments. Take the time to regulate your internal systems so you can move to a more comfortable place.

Be Mentally Engaged: Fit-in-Your-Life Exercises to Stretch Your Thinking

Choose a store, a market, or a restaurant with the intention of learning about a dish, a spice profile, or unique ingredients. Find a specialty or an ethnic market/restaurant and ask questions, explore new flavor combinations, discover new techniques, and learn from the *experts*. Learning by questioning activates multiple areas in your brain at the same time. You must use both basic sensory data and language processing as well as higher-level thinking skills to process, sort, categorize, and integrate the new information.

Add a challenge by defining one set of rules, but leave everything else open to interpretation. If you are cooking, write out your menu and take it—not a shopping list—to the store. You force yourself to think through the steps, formulate a plan to get everything you need, and problem-solve in the moment. Or if you are not cooking, pick a protein or a flavor profile and sort the menu using your predetermined criteria. Challenging yourself to be creative within a set of rules activates those areas of your brain that determine sequence, categories, and structure.

Amplify the experience by feeling everything.

Food is the perfect thing to *experience*. We so often eat because it is time or we *need* to eat. What a missed opportunity. Focus on how a food feels when it hits your tongue or the sensation that accompanies biting into something. Is it hot, cold, smooth, gritty, squishy, prickly, hard, gooey, spongy? Now focus on the taste. Is it sweet, bitter, savory, rich, sour, tangy, sparkly, spicy, complicated, creamy? How does it make you feel? Is it comforting, surprising, energizing, repulsive, offensive, warm?

As you know, adding a sensory experience to anything lights up each area of the brain that processes that sense and the areas that put those sensory experiences in context. Adding emotional value brings in those areas of the brain that process emotions and emotional memory.

Add more to your life. Live more fully. Process and think more intensively. Amplify and intensify your everyday experiences and you can turn them into brain workouts.

Be Mentally Engaged: Everyday Exercises

Practice triggering different emotions by looking at photographs. Go through an old photo album and think about what was happening in a specific photo. Take this exercise up another notch by sharing that experience with someone else. Describe as much of the scenario as you can, filling in emotional and sensory information.

When you can't go outside (like when you are working), bring the outside indoors and create a fuller sensory experience. Buy a plant or some flowers and vary the colors to trigger both sensory information processing and the sense of well-being that living things promote.

Turn on the soundtrack of nature—crashing waves, leaves rustling in the trees, birds singing and calling, water running over a rock. You can also buy a fountain, chimes, or a fan to create better, more peace-promoting sounds.

Surround yourself with colors that lift your spirits and make you feel good.

Put in your earbuds and listen to music that makes you feel good. Music can change your brain chemistry (much more on this later).

Light a scented candle, put out essential oils, or use fragrant flowers to trigger your sense of smell.

Experiment with your sense of touch and see what kinds of images and feelings you can create. Think about what happens when you:

- Wrap yourself in a warm blanket
- Pet a dog or cat
- Hold a comforting object like a stone or piece of jewelry and roll it around in your hands;
- Soak in a hot bath;
- Put on a piece of clothing that feels soft against your skin;
- Hold a piece of ice in your hand and feel it melt.

Take the time to close your eyes and picture a situation or place that feels peaceful and rejuvenating. As time allows, fill in those important things that elevate you and recharge your energy.

Stop during the day and capture a moment—make a mental description of every detail you find.

Focused Breathing

You will breathe from your diaphragm in this exercise and focus on the area underneath your rib cage feeling it move in and out. This will probably not feel natural at first, but this technique forms the basis

95

for most types of biofeedback and is a renewing and restoring form of breathing. A great way to redirect your thinking, this type of breathing clears your mind and resets your body's systems.

Breathe in through your nose, pushing your stomach out from your diaphragm. Feel the cool air as it enters through the nostrils. Focus on the feel of the air as it enters your body. Now let that air out through your mouth, completely emptying your lungs and pulling in at your diaphragm. Feel the warm air as it leaves your body. Repeat this, focusing on your breath only—feel the cool air on the way in and the warm air on the way out. Concentrate on moving your diaphragm out with the inhale and in with each exhale. Think about the pattern of your breathing. It is not necessarily even and steady, but has peaks and valleys. Continue this exercise, if comfortable for three minutes and repeat several times during the day.

This exercise, when done regularly, has been proven to help with concentration, relieve some kinds of headaches, and restore a balance in chemicals in the brain. In small doses, you will be able to restore a feeling of well-being and body balance.

Energizing Breath

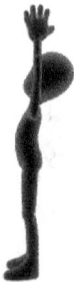

Stand up and take a deep breath. Bring your gaze upward as you breathe in. Move your arms above your head, touching your fingers together at the top.

Slowly release that breath, relax your neck, and allow your arms to gently glide down to your sides.

Let your eyes follow and pick a point on the horizon to rest your gaze.

Repeat this—breathe in, looking up, and raising your arms, and breathe out, gently relaxing your arms and neck, looking out at the horizon.

Now pick up the pace just a bit. Feel the air enter and exit your lungs. Feel your heart rate increase gradually as you increase the speed of the exercise. Repeat again, and this time feel the energy enter your body with each breath and a deep cleansing with each exhale. Stay in this exercise until you feel reenergized and renewed.

Devote today to something so daring even you can't believe you're doing it.

—Oprah Winfrey

CHAPTER EIGHT

Being Purposeful: How to Direct Your Life Toward Health

Do you see a simple pattern starting to emerge? Are you noticing how your body rewards you when you actively focus on those things that help you thrive?

When you amplify your daily experiences so that you feel more deeply, turn up the volume on your senses, and force yourself to think harder or differently, you nourish your brain with a healthy dose of chemicals and electricity. As you vary those activities and focus on stretching your thinking, you keep pathways in your brain open, active, and ready for use.

99

Keeping multiple pathways open makes it possible to process information in a variety of ways. So, if one route is blocked, your brain has options. You won't be left stuck in a problem you can't think your way through.

It's really pretty simple and straightforward. Ready for the next step?

Being purposeful takes this entire, simple model—one that moved from being active to being social and then to being mentally engaged—to the next level. Living a purpose-driven life fills in all the gaps in this everyday brain-health model.

Let's break down what living a purposeful life does for our brains and watch the pieces fall into place.

Finding and serving your purpose is, by nature, a multilayered process. You must think, evaluate, pull from prior experience and compare, look outside yourself, and choose to act. You have to go through the whole emotion-triggering process of figuring out what is important to you and why. Now take that another step further and move past understanding why this idea or action or train of thought is important to you to thinking about how you can make a difference and actually serve this purpose. Those are big, interconnected processes that tap into and force you to use many of your higher level thinking skills all at once, to find solutions and get you comfortable answers—ones that help you find productive pieces in an emotionally charged situation—to these big questions.

Being purposeful requires tapping into and engaging a deeply rooted emotional process that makes the parts of your brain work together in unique and interesting ways. That, in a nutshell, is what brain exercise should be.

This interconnected process, which forces a variety of cognitive processes to work together in harmony, fits perfectly into our brain-boosting line of thinking for a variety of reasons. The two big reasons stem from these facts. First, it is nearly impossible to be purposeful in a vacuum. And second, it is nearly impossible to live focused on your purpose and not be positive, solution-oriented, and optimistic.

Living and Sharing with a Positive Purpose

Think about it this way. Purposeful actions more times than not involve other people and situations that make you think outside yourself. Part of being purposeful means considering how your actions affect others and change a situation. Any time you reach out to others and make a connection, you feed your brain. Any time you do something that brings about a change, you trigger biological processes that will, in some form or another, also feed your brain.

Some of that comes from being social. Engaging in purposeful activities often allows you to connect with people who share an interest, a curiosity, or a passion. You might find that you expand your social circle in a positive way by building common ground and bonds with like-minded people. And you already know that when you join a group whose members support each other, it doubles your impact.

Some of that comes from being mentally active. You have to think and explore to get to the point where your purpose makes sense. Evaluating why something is important and finding a way to make a difference often requires learning new things and researching other points of view. That means engaging those higher-level thinking processes, and that activates those specific neural pathways.

Some of that comes from the mental engagement that simply happens when you imagine a better world. Your purpose often encompasses those things you can do to contribute to the world.

That means creating a picture or vision in your head to make it feel real and valid. Much of the planning portion of serving your purpose requires thinking about your personal impact and actually visualizing yourself making a difference.

101

That is strictly in your mind and something you may not practice in real life but it's effective to work through the details in your head beforehand. Living with a positive purpose takes you out of just getting through your days with nothing to remember and throws you squarely into engaging in your life.

Now consider this. Unlike any other "Be" we have discussed so far, "Be Purposeful" is not something a medical practitioner can write on a prescription pad for you to simply follow. If you are reading this book, you can, on some level, choose to be active, be social, and be engaged without making huge changes in your life or big shifts in perspective.

In most cases, being purposeful requires either a certain personality type or some major life adjustments. Unless being purposeful is an established pattern of behavior or part of who you are today, you can't just take a few minutes and be purposeful as a quick-hit method to improve brain health. It takes thought, soul searching, and strategic thinking, but is so worth the effort in many life- and health-enhancing ways.

Being focused on purpose and the positive requires conscious choices that last more than a second. It takes a solid belief that the long-term health and well-being benefits are worth all the work necessary to make those changes. The power of being positive and living a purposeful life can actually help you live better and more fully. There is proof that it is worth the effort. Once you make this way of living a habit, it takes less time and energy to focus on purpose.

Although not a magic pill that will reverse disease progression or prevent conditions from beginning, it is a way to approach life that will, without fail, help you deal with the bumps in the road better and more functionally.

Deeper Look at a View on Purpose and Meaning: Viktor Frankl

Let's look a branch of psychotherapy that rose out of the ashes of human tragedy, Logotherapy. Think about this chilling yet empowering fact: Viktor Frankl developed the foundations and techniques in a concentration camp in Nazi Germany. A whole branch of therapy and a philosophy grounded in the power to change your attitude and allow the intolerable and unthinkable to transform and elevate you rather than dismantle and destroy rose from Frankl's experience in two of Hitler's most notorious concentration camps, Auschwitz and Dachau.

Unlike scholars of his time (or even this time, for that matter), Frankl explains the what, the why, and the how of his perspective so perfectly that paraphrasing almost feels disrespectful.

Here, taken from his book *Man's Search for Meaning*, the basis of Frankl's approach to personal transformative thinking fits in so well with an everyday brain-health perspective:

> "Between stimulus and response, there is a space. In that space is our power to choose our response. In our response lies our growth and our freedom."

That way of thinking translates to this practical application also taken from the writings of Victor Frankl:

> "We can discover this meaning in life in three different ways: 1) by creating a work or doing a deed; 2) by experiencing something or encountering someone; and 3) by the attitude we take toward unavoidable suffering."

The Science Behind Being Purposeful

Several factors make it so difficult to bring such variable human elements into the laboratory and make statements based on those studies that generalize to everyday life. But primarily, testing the effects of being purposeful and positive on brain health is difficult because it is so hard to isolate those two traits and separate their effect from other healthy activities and behaviors.

However, some mounting and convincing evidence, both anecdotal and from the laboratory, supports the overall health-boosting benefits of living a life driven by a purpose. Study after study indicates that, in a variety of conditions from diabetes to addiction recovery to heart disease and more, positive connections form between one's health and feeling purposeful. Results show that the belief that life has meaning empowers people to heal quicker and remain healthy longer. Outcomes are better across the board.

Brain health, in particular, is harder to isolate. Here is something to think about from the highly publicized Rush Memory and Aging Project's long-term studies on changes in cognition and quality of thinking as people age. Preliminary results (2006, 2008, 2009, 2010) indicated that there was a tie between feeling positive and purposeful and lower rates of cognitive decline. Those with rosier outlooks who felt like they were living a purposeful life stayed sharper longer. The Rush research team took that a step further and tried to isolate these factors a bit more. In a study published in 2012 with more controlled variables, they concluded:

> "Higher levels of purpose in life reduce the deleterious effects of AD pathologic changes on cognition in advanced age." (Boyle, et al, 2012)

Just think about what that means. People with the same type of changes in their brains had differing levels and rates of cognitive decline that could be tied, at least in part, to *feeling purposeful*. These are people with similar biological markers and in similar stages of disease progression, yet the group that reported "higher levels of purpose" on a standard measure had fewer thinking problems than those who reported "lower levels of purpose" on that same scale.

Could it really be that living a positive, purposeful life can help you protect your brain and help fight the symptoms of Alzheimer's disease and reduce your chances of cognitive decline where Alzheimer's is not present? This summarizes some of the general findings from that study.

Researchers tested subjects for seven years and found those participants who expressed a sense of purpose were, when compared with people who expressed no sense of purpose in life were:

- More than 50 percent less likely to develop symptoms associated with Alzheimer's disease
- Two-and-a-half times more likely not to exhibit signs of dementia
- Almost a third less likely to develop mild cognitive impairment—impairment that is below normal but does not hinder daily activity

One study, even a longitudinal study with great controls, is not enough to draw any sweeping conclusions, but it does point us in a good direction and fills in some of the color in the everyday brain-health picture.

Being Purposeful and Positive Psychology

Let's now take this a step further and look at a few theories about why this might work and how it ties to brain function.

Positive Psychology is an emerging and compelling branch of psychology, particularly when evaluating benefits of living a purposeful life. According to the University of Pennsylvania Positive Psychology Center:

> "Positive Psychology is the scientific study of the strengths and virtues that enable individuals and communities to thrive. The field is founded on the belief that people want to lead meaningful and fulfilling lives, to cultivate what is best within themselves, and to enhance their experiences of love, work, and play."

Positive psychology takes the study of human behavior and moves it to a wellness-promoting model. It focuses on what you can to do to be more resilient, healthier, and better able to thrive.

From research in positive psychology comes a body of work that focuses on experiential living. These studies and their findings are particularly interesting when working to better understand everyday brain health.

An early study in the field found that when people engage in an experience that connects them on a deep level—feeling in the *flow,* where time and space seem to disappear—they are so gratified they want to replicate that feeling. They wish to do this not for any tangible reward they will get out of doing so, but just for the feeling. The activity becomes its own reward not only because they are so fully engaged in the moment, but because it feeds something deeper in them and they want to repeat it simply to get that connected feeling. Isn't that fascinating?

The other compelling set of findings in positive psychology deals with inspiring others to be purposeful. Researchers found that watching others perform acts of kindness and behave altruistically spurred more activity. You can inspire others to live more selflessly just by being selfless and modeling that behavior. That is pretty cool.

Be Purposeful in Perspective

Think about this: What if having a reason to get out of bed in the morning ultimately gave you more mornings to get out of bed—or better days to spend once you were up? What if simple shifts in attitude, perspective, and focus could make that much of a difference in your life? And what if the really cool part was that there is no downside?

When you feel purposeful, you are more optimistic, hopeful, and have more of a positive outlook on life. Some positive psychologists suggest that even small things, like positive self-talk, can turn on cell activity in your brain.

Beyond that, those looking at the effects of being positive have found that this approach may actually strengthen your immune system's response to disease and allow you to heal faster.

Even though we don't totally understand why or how the underlying mechanisms work, like in so many other cases, the information that we do have is enough to act on.

The idea of being positive and purposeful doesn't carry any warning labels because no studies, in the laboratory or observational, document any adverse effects of being purposeful or positive. If we take that information along with evidence that living a fulfilling and purposeful life promote health and longevity, and delays some thinking issues, why not embrace this approach to life?

I heard a *TED Talk* presented by Dr. Martin Seligman, the leading mind in positive psychology and an inspirational leader in the field. His perspective is this: Psychology and psychiatry have made enormous breakthroughs to helping people feel better. That is great, but when an entire field of study focuses squarely on treating disease and alleviating misery, something huge is missing. He proposes that we look at *normal* lives and making people who are not troubled even happier, more functional, and more productive. He believes psychology historically has overlooked creating intervention and protocols to make people happier rather than simply less miserable. Those are such compelling thoughts and worth digging into to see where they might take psychology and neuroscience.

Right now researchers across the world are studying the neuroscience behind all of this and looking for interventions that will help people find that bit of purpose and use it to create a better life. From the neurochemistry of altruism to finding meaning by getting in the flow, real science seeks to unlock some of the mysteries behind why meaning and purpose create changes in the brain—and possibly helps people live and think better.

Brain Injury Insights

Some odd, unexplained side effects occur after any major brain change, and one of the strangest and most universal is apathy.

I still have not found any research that goes beyond acknowledging apathy as a common condition post-brain trauma but, across the board, every single person I have spoken to with conditions ranging from MS to chemo-brain to TBI caused by explosions, talks about periods of not being able to find meaning in life. They describe simply not caring. Although it sounds like depression, it is—plain and simple—apathy.

This was not only a major personality change for me, but also a change in how I chose to live my life. My life was in my head and everything I encountered was about what I felt. It is difficult to live with purpose or find meaning when life becomes confined within the walls of your cranium.

How I dealt with my own apathy defined my path to recovery. In one of the rare moments when I did care, I made a conscious decision to force a focus change and practice my formerly highly developed empathy skills. I created an exercise that made me pick a person and try to see the world through their eyes. I started at home attempting to look at the world through my husband's and my son's eyes. I then worked my way out into the world, first with my mother and then to less safe, more foreign perspectives. This became part of my daily routine and led me deeper into my recovery than any other exercise in my repertoire.

It sounds odd that practicing empathy can take you out of your fog, but I can tell you from personal experience that it can. Practicing shifting my perspective and pushing beyond what I saw in my head absolutely escalated my healing. I felt it working and it gave me confidence.

～

Practicing empathy helps us find meaning, and although not yet proven, could also help build a better brain.

Those with progressive brain diseases, ones where the goal is to keep progression at bay and treat the symptoms, often lose hope. I can't help but think that some branch of therapy—some way to practice empathy—holds the power to make two thing happen.

First, practicing empathy serves as a distraction and can keep you from falling down the rabbit hole of apathy (that turns apathy to despair). It can move you to a place bigger than yourself. Open up the world to look beyond disease progression and live in this moment.

Second, seeing the world through someone else's eyes provides a glimpse at the depth of human perspective out there. There are lives that are worse and lives that are better, but also there are lives not defined by a diagnosis. That provides a bit of light and, in some cases, confidence. We know that changing your view makes you *feel*, and that fires up activity in your brain.

Be Purposeful: Roll-in-Your-Life Perspective Shifts

So how can you live with more purpose and feel more fulfilled? When you look at the kind of shifts and pivots you need to make in order to be purposeful, you must make a big change in attitudinal focus. Give these concrete shifts in attitude a shot.

When evaluating where you are and what you are doing, put the emphasis on your strengths instead of what needs to be fixed. By looking at yourself in the context of situation and focusing on your positive qualities, you put yourself in a powerfully empathetic position. Take that a step further and look closely at those strengths. See how you can use them to support, evaluate, fill in gaps, or help find a solution when one is needed. It may seem simple and logical, but that can be a big shift in thinking.

Or try this: Change where you focus your attention. Although we don't necessarily know why, we become fascinated by the negative. Even when we take stock of the people around us, we tend to look at those who are down to some degree. Yes, that can help you build empathy, but it can also give you a skewed view of the world. Instead of focusing on unhappy people, actively seek out and look for *fulfilled* people. See if you can figure out what makes them more positive. What are they doing differently? When you identify those traits, work on rolling them into your own life. You may be surprised at how far you will take not just your life, but also how many others you inspire to be fulfilled as well. Make simple shifts in what you observe and emulate.

Or try this: Look more deeply inside yourself—how your body works, the tools you use to be productive, your daily activities, and how you use those things to be successful. Shift the focus to fit engaging, meaningful activities in your life to best support your success. Can you make some changes in perspective so that your daily activities help you serve your purpose? What changes will help you refocus your daily life and move you toward finding and living with more meaning?

Be Purposeful: Roll-in-Your-Life Activities

You can set yourself on a purposeful path to a life filled with more meaning (and better brain health) by paying attention to what you already do each day, look more closely, and make necessary shifts.

Carry a notebook and pen in your pocket. As you live your life, note those things you really care about. What makes you feel on a deeper level? What gives you that little jolt of excitement or joy? Write down all the moments, big and small, no matter how quickly they pass. Take a few minutes at the end of the day to review that list. You might find items on the list seemed more meaningful at the time might have completely slipped through the maze that filters memory. If you had not written them down, they may have been lost to the rest of the day. Bringing into focus what makes you feel will help you zero in on finding meaningful activities. That way you can figure out how to amplify them, make them happen more regularly, and carve out a permanent place for purpose in your daily activities.

Once you have that list, look for similarities within the entries. Is there a common theme? What you were physically doing? Who were you with? Where were you? Are there other factors that seem to repeat? Then sort your list into categories according to commonalities.

Carry that refined list with you the next day. Think about those categories as you go through your routine. Did your themes repeat? Put some kind of note or mark next to that category. Did you notice something you might have missed before? Think of your list as a work in progress and add any new items in the proper categories. Do any things fall outside a category? Create a space for them and look at them later. A new category might pop up. Repeat the categorizing and sorting activity at the end of day two. Take a minute to think about how your focus differed.

Repeat this for a few days. When your categories and lists feel fairly inclusive, review what you have done. Take those qualities that gave you the most joy and create a separate list. Now create a plan to focus more on taking items from those categories—the ones that make you smile and give you joy—and incorporate them into even more parts of your life. For example, if one of your categories is food, find a way to make food purposeful. Teach someone to cook or cook with someone who lives alone. Take a meal to someone who is feeling down, or take that person out to lunch. We all must eat so why not make it a purposeful activity?

Ask yourself these questions: Can you refocus your day or retool parts of your life to emphasize those meaningful items? How can you tailor your daily activities and refocus all those things you to do to successfully get from morning to night, to include more moments that give you joy? It does not have to be a big change but recentering, refocusing, and reworking your routine to fit in more meaning.

Be Purposeful: Dream Big

When you make big shifts in your life, you need a place to start. Filling your life with more meaning by making little shifts and focusing on finding purpose and joy helps, but if you want to change how you live your life and how you make big decisions, it helps to set up the building blocks.

Sometimes that means learning a new process. In this case, you might need to learn how to dream. It sounds odd, but we have been taught to temper our dreams and choose what the world or others around us find appropriate. Here's a description of the process and followed by an example.

Dreaming With a Purpose: The Process

Get a brand new notebook. Before you write anything, make sure you create an organized way to record 1) the date you wrote each entry; 2) a description of the dream (why it is important to you); and 3) notes along the way. All are important, and you don't want to lose any details because you did not plan ahead. Each dream will have its own page(s), so each of the items could have its own line or you might want to create headings across the top of the page. Do whatever works best for you.

Sit in a place where you feel inspired and away from distractions. Close your eyes and imagine yourself completely and thoroughly relaxed and at peace. Dreaming requires letting go and that is not an easy task. Dreams that support your goal of finding meaning and purpose require you to be alone with your thoughts. These are your dreams, not the dreams others have for you.

Now imagine feeling fulfilled—feeling that your life has meaning and purpose. Search for something you can describe in time and space, where you can see yourself active and engaged.

Once you have something clearly in mind, record the date and describe, in as much detail as you need, what you see and why all that is in that scene is important to you. When you go back and reread this part, it should feel significant.

Look at your current life. Think about how far you need to travel to get to this fulfilled place and start mapping out a plan. Set goals to get you closer and closer to that fulfilled place. Follow the standard goal-setting mantra. Each goal is something that is very specific, measurable (you must be able to tell you are there), achievable (it must be possible), realistically high (don't set the bar too low or too high), and must have a time limit. When you set goals that support purposeful dreaming, you must add two more vital criteria. First, make sure that the goal helps you get to the specific dream and that the dream fills a purposeful need in your life and fits your core values. Second, make sure each goal is meaningful to you. Is your goal a way to move you closer to leading a life full of meaning for you or is this something you think you should do? Check and double check each goal.

Dreaming With a Purpose: An Example

A long time ago I determined that mentoring fed this part of me that I could not describe or understand. I knew watching others succeed as a result of something I set in motion charged me up, lifted my spirits, and allowed me the confidence to do things I did not believe I could. My accident did not knock this out of me; it just changed its focus.

Post-brain injury my purposeful dream turned into this: I want to empower those who feel hopeless after a brain trauma. I want to help them find a way to lift themselves up and live a better, richer, fuller life than they imagine they possibly could have. I want to spread the message that by turning up the volume on life, almost anyone can think better, live better, and, by example, inspire others to do the same. These are not small dreams and they certainly have very little structure.

To make them a reality, I had to write out a plan that included detailed steps toward that goal, in a much-abbreviated form, it went something like this:

- Get an advanced degree
- Start working in the field and get some direct experience

- Develop some tools
- Test those tools and rework them
- Build a website
- Build an audience, credibility, and a tribe
- Expand and adapt with new knowledge and research
- Create a place (or two) like a book, a blog, and website to start spreading the word
- Practice what I preach every day

Make a plan to be purposeful every single day of your life and feel the rewards every single day of your life!

Do not overlook tiny good actions, thinking they are of no benefit; even tiny drops of water in the end will fill a huge vessel.

—Buddha

CHAPTER NINE

Being Complicated: How to Amplify Your Life

It's time to take an even bigger leap and consider creating a new life pattern and a retooled perspective—one that turns up the volume on your life and truly fires your brain on multiple levels. What we are really talking about here is rolling a set of habits that integrate more than one way of "Being" into one activity. By doing that, you are increasing your impact, maximizing your efforts, and amplifying your daily experiences.

In this section we will first consider how to combine the Be's of brain health as outlined in the previous sections. Then we will take a

117

closer look at a life enhancing activity, music, and examine how you can use music to boost your brain power by activating so much more.

Pretty powerful stuff and, yes, another conscious shift in perspective and how you approach your life, but one that will expand how you behave and think about your daily activities.

Challenge Yourself to Be Complicated.

When you accept the challenge and embrace the idea of being complicated, you are taking the necessary steps to heal, bolster, and fortify your brain in the most powerful ways. As an added bonus, you will rev up the quality of your life and enhancing your daily experiences. This, without question, is a situation where you simply win.

Be Complicated: Double Your Impact

Sometimes a simple change can make a big difference. Adding new elements to your daily brain-healthy activities brings a whole new dimension to transforming everyday activities into brain-healthy life boosters. Let's look at a few examples.

Consciously Be Active and Engaged
While Out and About

When you are out for a walk, you can add fire up some additional pathways in your brain by making a few small changes or simple additions. Try these things:

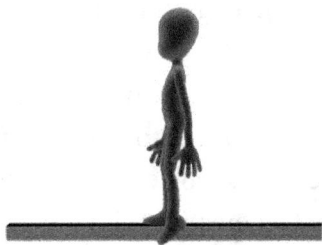

When on a side street, choose to walk on the curb instead of the sidewalk. This will force you to think about keeping your balance and intentionally placing one foot in front of the other. And that kicks in at least two more brain processes.

Change your shoes. Try round bottomed sneakers, hiking boots, or sandals instead of athletic shoes. Just by changing your shoes, you add a bit of a challenge. You change your experience and make the simple act of getting from one place to the next a more complicated task. Make your brain work just a bit harder or in a different way, and you will reap the rewards.

Listen to an audiobook or a podcast. Let your mind go in more than one direction, feed your imagination, or learn something new while you maximize not only how you use your time but also how you activate your thinking processes. When you force yourself to take on this kind of complicated activity, the benefits multiply.

Go to the gym with a friend and have a deep conversation as part of your workout. Try to see the conversation from your friend's point of view. Your brain must work hard to coordinate movements, follow the conversation, and be engaged. By shifting your focus and look at the world through the eyes of another, you also practice your empathy skills.

Consciously Be Active, Be Engaged, and Be Social and.... It's All About Dinner.

Take something you do every day and figure out how to amplify the effects. Here's a concrete example of how to make this happen.

119

Everyone has to eat, so why not try this: Choose a group of people with whom you enjoy spending time with and plan an interactive meal. Have each person bring a set of ingredients to go with a particular theme. You supply the main ingredient (the protein and any other central items) and the theme (farm to table, Moroccan, organic, comfort food, etc.). Have each guest bring at least one spice or herb and another ingredients that go with the theme. Get creative with the instructions and give guests as much or as little direction as you want. The group will cook the meal using every ingredient available. Focus on each ingredient, both as you cook and as you eat. Talk about what goes together and what doesn't. Try a few experiments and see how they blend. Most importantly, include everyone in the active part of cooking. That way this becomes a complicated group brain workout.

How about another exercise? No time to plan a party? Shop at a farmers' market as a way to get active and engaged with your ingredients in a highly social environment. Arrive with no plan and no menu so that you are better able to explore all the options available to you. It is easy to overlook something amazing if you walk in with an agenda, so let yourself create as you go.

Ask the vendors questions about their products. Find out about growing seasons and what weather conditions might change the flavor or the availability of that product. Ask what spices and herbs complement it and be sure to ask vendors their favorite ways to use it and if they can share a favorite recipe. Take it all in, create a menu, buy the ingredients, go home, cook, and savor the flavors.

Live in an area where farmers' markets are seasonal and you are not in season? Pick an area of town that has a distinct population and try the same thing at an ethnic market. When you find a Greek deli or an Indian or South African market, you tune in to the unfamiliar, wake up your senses, and allow yourself to feed your curiosity and be more creative.

Consciously Be Active, Be Social, Be Purposeful, and Be Engaged: Active Volunteering

Do you have a cause that sparks a passion or interest in you? Find something that you love and dive in just a bit deeper.

There are some easy and effective ways to increase the impact of your brain-boosting activity.

For example, are you interested in the environment? See if there are nonprofits or service organizations in your area that focus on the environment. Go to their websites and search for events that fit into your life. Sign up for a clean-up or beautification project. Volunteer at a fundraising event.

Can you walk or run? Races for causes take place everywhere and require very little extra on your part because everything is organized. In most cases, all you have to do is show up and reap the brain benefits of being active, purposeful, and social. Your small effort makes a huge difference for both yourself and the cause, so everyone wins. You can increase that impact even more by forming or joining a team, all walking or running together.

Love to travel and want to make a difference? Search volunteer vacations and see what pops up. Find a match, do your research, and pack your bag!

Love to travel and passionate about learning? Check out cooking schools or trips sponsored by universities, groups like National Geographic. If you are over 60, check out Road Scholars. Some of these trips take place in locations where you can participate (experiential learning) and others include classroom learning (mini-universities). Find a topic that sparks your passion and learn more from the experts in a social setting.

Consciously Be Engaged and Be Purposeful With a Citizen Science Project

Does astronomy, plants, animals, conservation, teaching, or community building excite you? Check out a citizen science project and get involved on an even more meaningful level. Citizen scientists are non-scientists, non-specialists who collect data to add to the body of scientific knowledge. There are a ton of projects out there.

It is so rewarding when the goals and values of a project match your own. Personally, I love the philosophy of one specific project, the Marine Animal Identification Network. This project tracks seals and participants report information about migration. This statement sums it all up for me:

> "In many cases, we learn through the imprecise science of serendipity whereby a matrix of possibilities results in a report: the right person in the right place at the right time knowing the right person to contact."

How wonderful is it that any of us, just by chance, can be that person at the right place at the right time who can make a valuable contribution to science?

It is surprisingly easy to find projects that require very little investment of time or technology. All you really need is a smartphone or computer and a few extra minutes to participate in some of these projects! Search for citizen science projects in a geographic area or that have to do with a specific interest.

Love the outdoors? Check out the National Wildlife Federation for a diverse list of projects, from backyard birders to butterfly counting to star gazing.

Or you can work with the Audubon Society's Rivers Project through the Office of the U.S. Army Corps of Engineers and the Cornell Lab of Ornithology. They monitor and track birds in the bottom-land forests on the Mississippi River. Observe, record, report, contribute!

How about working with NASA from your own backyard? NASA has several citizen science projects going on now, with more to come.

These projects are so cool because they give you an opportunity to learn and grow personally while helping a field of research.

The key is to look for those opportunities that will help you feed your passion, be active (get out and do something), and meet new people. You might not only fill some gaps in your quest to serve your purpose, but you might also find like-minded people working on other projects that will fuel you in other ways. Often finding one project leads to another, which may lead you to try new things and push the limits of your comfort zone.

Be Complicated: Music

Music is a powerful brain drug—one that can be used to fortify you, keep you balanced, and build up that healthy reserve you need to thrive. Music fills your life and fuels your brain like nothing else.

Think about this. Music engages your senses, triggers memories, and fires emotions. It can help you look at life through a different lens and can actually change the way you feel about something. How many times have you put on music to lift your mood or change your outlook? How many passive activities—just sit back and listen—can do that for you? Now that is real power.

Add to that the fact that listening to music makes you want to move, activates your imagination, sparks emotions, forces you to find patterns and harmony, and triggers all of those language and meaning processes in your brain. Music becomes a truly *complicated* activity that hits you on so many levels. When you put music in perspective and look at its benefits through an everyday brain health-lens, you are, at the very minimum, active, engaged, and triggering emotions. In many cases, music is also social and helps you find meaning. Seriously, music can hit it all—Be Active, Be Social, Be Engaged, Be Purposeful.

A quick look at the science behind how your brain processes music will help you understand its complicated nature and just how much it can do to change the quality of your thinking and your life.

The Science Behind Music and the Brain

The study of music's effects on the brain is a hotly researched topic. Right now, neuroscientists are mapping, very specifically, what happens in the body and the brain when you listen to music, why it happens, and ways to capitalize on those things to bring about change.

Technology opened up a whole new area in the study of music and the brain. Relatively new research is examining how the brain processes different parts of music and how each looks in an active brain.

Among the many findings, a few stand out and are particularly important to understanding how this complicated activity can fire up so many areas of the brain and encourage cooperative efforts between and among brain processes.

Researchers found that brains process music in almost an identical way, regardless of a person's musical tastes, age, or educational level. Studies show, music consistently lit up those regions that regulate movement, planning, attention, and memory. That means when you listen to music, you are involved in a much more meaningful process than just processing sound. This process represents a true collaboration in the brain filled with organized, multi-layered, and repetitive sets of sensory experiences—all things that our brains just love.

So if the process is the same, why do some people like opera and others like grunge rock? Interestingly, the other areas of the brain that light on fire while listening to music are those responsible for emotions and emotional memory. Your brain constantly compares what you liked before—the rhythm, the melody, the harmony, and the tonal qualities—to what you're listening to now. It decides how to process the piece of music emotionally. Vast and varied brain activation.

Music as a Tool: Music Therapy

There is little doubt that music can heal and help change the way you think and process information. Music has the power to help you rewrite the stories of your life just by making you feel and experience more deeply. Music therapy works for a variety of reasons but mostly because the brain and body both respond to melody, lyrics, and rhythms, as described above, on not just a physical level but also an emotional level. Beyond that, music often evokes memories bound to time, geography, and biography.

Listening to and getting involved in music activates all those areas of the brain that control physical and emotional responses plus those that process memories, geography, and life events. That is a lot happening from just one activity.

There are, without question, measurable, positive changes in brain activity and blood flow when simply thinking about music. I could talk about the chemical and electrical changes in every single area of the brain associated with higher-level functioning, problem solving, creativity, and emotion. Add to that the therapeutic effects of learning how to play a musical instrument, and music just may hold the key to tapping into and maintaining a healthy brain.

Insights from Brain Injury

Music was an integral part of my own recovery, and I still use it daily to restore, renew, and rebuild.

I am not alone in this. The following powerful story describes how music changed the experience of MS for a valued colleague of mine.

"When I was first diagnosed with MS in 1992, music truly came to my rescue and its healing power became undeniable. When I was first diagnosed, I was hospitalized for five days, in hopes the steroid infusions and break from the everyday baloney of daily living and caring for my three young daughters—then 9, 8, 6—would help me walk again, see clearly again. My first day or two in the hospital, my older brother visited and brought along a Walkman. He told me to just shut out the world by putting on the headphones, closing my eyes, and listening to music that soothes me, whatever genre that may be. I can't recall exactly what I listened to, but I kept those headphones on throughout the hospital stay, removing them only when my family or other visitors came or doctors needed me to interact with them. I even slept with the headphones on. No TV, no reading—nothing but music. I have no doubt whatsoever that the Walkman saved my sanity, quelled my fears, helped me walk again—something the doctors were not confident I would be able to do.

Since then, music has been a huge part of my recovery process. To me, there's something endlessly comforting in certain compositions like George Winston's work. Music truly does soothe the savage beast, and his piano tunes soothe and heal me like nothing else. I hadn't listened to him in many years as I'd been doing okay, but when I recently faced challenges like never before, I pulled out all the George Winston music we own, filled the five-CD Bose, and blasted it

126

throughout the house for days on end, hoping it would work as magically as it did for many years. It helped, no doubt. I even mentioned to my middle daughter when she called once and wondered why the music was so loud that I was trying to reformat my brain with George Winston. She understood because she had witnessed the magic when I was first diagnosed.

George Winston isn't the only music that saves me, though. I have music playing in the background every day, most of the day. Some days it's alternative rock, others it's classic rock, and more often now than in days past it's pop—because it's so darn easy to sing to. And as you know, singing to it makes a difference in the brain.

Music makes a difference for me when I have to get through scary spots, and the process of this disease has some scary spots. There are particular songs that I believe literally saved me from hysteria at my most scary medical moments: specifically, getting through an MRI when my claustrophobia has gotten worse; helping me maintain composure on the way to hear how bad that MRI was as well as the course of action to take; helping me maintain peace and positivity after learning how compromised my brain has become.

On days where I feel like I am losing who I am to MS, I use music to step closer back to being me. I watch videos with lyrics and sing along. There are times when I'm doing such that I honestly feel a shift in my brain, a soothing clarity, and a positivity that sticks with me along with the earworm after viewing."

Even though our experiences are all so different, we share one thing—a brain that guides our actions, our decisions, our physiology, our emotions, and the quality of our lives. We hold the power to heal ourselves and build better brains. How empowering is that?

I have no doubt that even though the jury is still out on many findings that will lead us to understanding all the workings of the brain. But we already have the means to harness the unimaginable power of our brains to heal ourselves and move our lives in a different direction—just by thinking, doing, and being.

It's not the load that breaks you down, it's the way you carry it.

– Lena Horne

CHAPTER TEN

Being Powerful: If I Could Do This, So Can You

On my path to *Okay* and through my studies and life's work that followed, I learned how to use the power of the brain to heal itself and grow new cells as a tool to a better quality of life. Not just cognitive life, but life in general. I learned how to maximize brain functioning by amplifying my life and paying attention to both my body and my surroundings. I learned that many things could be changed—even the functioning of my brain—if I made basic shifts and altered my perspective. I learned that neuroplasticity, the power of the brain to rebuild and rewire, is a powerful thing which can actually be directed. That knowledge changed my life and it can change yours.

Recognizing the Signs

The real complicating factor is this: We are not trained to recognize what is happening in our own lives or in others' lives and that blind spot keeps us from understanding what and how to change.

We simply don't see, recognize, or understand the challenges and how they come to light in everyday life. It is so important to know what you are facing and how to react to best support recovery.

On my path I discovered the way, a few truths and some misconceptions and each has changed how I view my personal challenges and those I see for others.

Insight No. 1: Just because someone looks fine does not mean they see you or understand what the hell is coming out of your mouth. Neither speaking loudly nor enunciating more clearly helps clarify anything. It's probably not a hearing issue. When someone doesn't understand, take the time to figure out how to reframe your comment or phrasing.

Insight No. 2: Personality changes after a brain injury are inevitable. When interacting with someone with a brain injury, don't expect that person to act like they used to—it is both unfair and unrealistic. Change the way you relate to them, at least until they can get their feet planted on the ground. Know that this personality change is neither easy nor comfortable for the person experiencing it either. It is much easier for you to change your reactions than to expect change. It is as though you are steering a precision racecar, able to easily turn on a dime, while they struggle to steer an ocean liner.

Insight No. 3: Never tell anyone it is okay to settle. That is a choice no one should ever make for anyone else. No one has the right to rewrite our scripts–even when things go wrong. Never take away someone's power to make choices and reach for more.

Insight No. 4: Brain rebuilding requires a bit of anger to fuel the fire. This especially happens during those times when it doesn't feel worth it to continue to be patient and persistent. Allow the injured party to be angry. The trick is to help him or her embrace and use that anger in a productive way.

Finding the Right Combination

A few universal ideas and attitudes will help you move to the next level—whatever that is—but realistically there is no magic combination of activities and exercises that work for everyone. Finding that right combination, that set of activities that will allow you to enjoy your life while building a stronger, more resilient brain is critical.

Think about this: You have the power to change how you think and act. Those behavior changes can help you change how well your brain works on both a functional and a structural level. That is real power, real hope, and your best real-world solution.

The Biggest Lesson of All and What it Means for You

My road to *Okay* taught me that we all have the power to heal ourselves by thinking, acting, and doing. That is huge! And so empowering.

I learned that even though the process is not always easy, it can be rewarding, fulfilling, and oh so worth it.

I pushed life until it pushed me down. Each and every time it did, I tried hard to get up and start where I left off before the stumble. Even though shaking off the fall and rubbing the injuries was not fair nor pleasant, it was exactly what needed to happen if I was going to move to a place where I was thinking clearly enough to make a difference. I was and still am driven to use this detour on my life's path to create something we can all use as a guide to live each day better and more fully, regardless of our individual stories.

133

I knew that the only way I was going to do that was to keep getting up and challenging myself and my expanding my world. I could not settle for or get comfortable with less than I wanted. I had to pay attention to the details about what was working and what was not, and then focus on how each of those things made me feel. I was determined to figure out why that was—the science, the logic, and the motivations behind it all. I needed to record it all and make it make sense as I did the work.

During my recovery and well into the current building, maximizing, and amplifying phase of my life, I saw the need to tell the whole story of brain health—from function to biology and chemistry, to neuroplasticity and rebuilding, and finally, to hope.

My storyline, my script must include a section that maximizes what I learned and allows me to share that in a form that is useful, practical, and implementable for others.

Staying "down" was not a long-term option for me if I wanted to live without compromise.

As I rebuilt my brain, I retooled my life and came out on the other side healthier, more productive, more satisfied, and so much more in tune with myself—mind, body, and soul. The gift I found at the bottom of that paper bag was that I could share all of this with you.

Acknowledgements

I am incredibly grateful to Lois Alter Mark, Lisa Carpenter, and Terri Pilot. Thank you for your guidance, encouragement, and honesty, and for sharing your expertise and wisdom. I am also grateful to Michael Mark for pushing me to write my story—even when I dug in my heels and resisted. Repeatedly. You made this piece of work so much more relevant and valuable. Thanks to Terrence Spohn for taking the project apart and putting it all back together in an order that made so much more sense.

I owe huge thank yous to Elin Waldal, Helene Bludman, Jackie Combs, Kathie Moore, Cathy Chester, Katie O'Brasky, Judi Bonilla, Patricia Patton, and Karen Austin for reading, advising, sharing stories, and encouraging me. Thank you to all those who generously shared their oh so personal stories with me and allowed me to share them.

Last but not least, thank you to my husband Dan for standing by me through all my self-doubt and the huge learning curve of writing this piece. Words simply don't say enough.

Note About References

I used more than 150 journal articles and books, both scholarly and mainstream, to create this book and to develop my approach. If you would like a reference list or more information on any particular reference or fact in the text, send me an email and I will send you what you require. ruth@rollingmulliganpublishing.com

Gratefully,

Ruth Curran, MS